Run for Your Life

A Book for Beginning Women Runners

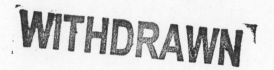

Run for Your Life

A Book for Beginning Women Runners

Deborah Reber

A Perigee Book

A Perigee Book
Published by The Berkley Publishing Group
A division of Penguin Putnam Inc.
375 Hudson Street
New York, New York 10014

Copyright © 2002 by Deborah Reber
Text design by Tiffany Kukec
Illustrations by Michele Reber
Cover design by Charles Björklund and Wendy Bass
Cover photo of woman stretching: Superstock
Cover photo of woman eating fruit: Anton Vengo/Superstock
Cover photo of woman drinking water: Superstock
Cover photo of woman running: Superstock
Author photo by Suzanne Karp Photography

First edition: April 2002
Published simultaneously in Canada.

Visit our website at www.penguinputnam.com

Library of Congress Cataloging-in-Publication Data

Reber, Deborah.
Run for your life : a book for beginning women runners / Deborah Reber.
p.   cm.
ISBN 0-399-52756-7
1. Running for women.   I. Title.

GV1061.18.W66 R43   2002
796.42'082—dc21
2001053106

Printed in the United States of America

10   9   8   7   6   5   4   3   2   1

Every effort has been made to ensure that the information contained in this book is complete and accurate. However, neither the publisher nor the author is engaged in rendering professional advice or services to the individual reader. The ideas, procedures, and suggestions contained in this book are not intended as a substitute for consulting with your physician. All matters regarding your health require medical supervision. Neither the author nor the publisher shall be liable or responsible for any loss, injury or damage allegedly arising from any information or suggestion in this book.

To Derin, my running partner for life

Contents

Foreword

I began running in the '70s. I was in my thirties, with two small children. I grew up in the '50s and '60s when physical activity for women consisted of chasing the kids and cleaning the house. Normal women didn't sweat . . . or run . . . or enter races.

By the mid-'70s, women were testing their wings. Running provided the perfect way to fly; we didn't need expensive equipment—just a decent pair of running shoes, old shorts and a T-shirt, and the will to take the first steps out the door. I took those first steps and never looked back. I am proud to be a runner . . . a woman runner.

I wore men's shorts and T-shirts and a maternity bra for support. I began my running career in tennis shoes and then graduated to women's running shoes, which had recently become available—it was paradise.

I was an oddity, running the roads with not a drop of self-consciousness. People stared. I proudly met their gaze. As my mileage increased, so did my self-confidence. The laughing-stock of gym class was now an athlete.

Races in the early days were no-frills events, unlike the mega-races of today. Equal awards for men and women were unheard of. Those of us who commented about the disparity were called "Women's Libbers."

How far women's running has come since those early days. We now have state-of-the-art shoes and clothes and equitable age groups and prizes in road races. We are role models for young women. We revel in the power of our bodies.

Some of my happiest running memories have been the times I have run and raced with my daughter, Marcy. Running provides an intense bonding experience for women. Whether as part of a training group or a mom-daughter duo, the close-ness is like no other.

My Running 101 course consisted of figuring things out on my own or asking a lot of questions (usually of men). Deborah Reber's wonderful book, *Run for Your Life*, provides all the information I wish was available to me when I began to run. It's written in a light, easy-to-follow style with lots of personal anecdotes. When I finished the book, I felt as if I had gained a new running friend.

Fledgling runners, especially women, need encouragement. Feel like you're not making progress? This book will help you understand the improvement curve. Feel uncomfortable run-ning alone? Check the information on running safety. Thinking about running your first race? Deborah will point you to the starting line. What to do if the call of nature occurs on a run? Not to worry. That's covered, too. What about running in snow or rain? Running is a year-round activity and this book will show you the way.

Run for Your Life is peppered with quotes from women runners of all ages. Their enthusiasm is contagious. Read them again when you need an extra dollop of motivation. The resource pages provide a plethora of helpful information. Is this a book you will refer to again and again? Without a doubt. Whether you're a beginning runner or a seasoned vet like me, *Run for Your Life* is a book that's like an old and trusted friend. Keep it handy. You'll want to rely on this friend for years to come.

Freddi Carlip,

president, Road Runners Club of America

editor/publisher, *Runner's Gazette*

July 2001

Introduction

There is a movement gaining strength among women. I'm not talking about the "women's movement" or the Equal Rights Amendment. It's something much larger, more inclusive and much more powerful. As we enter the twenty-first century, women are finally starting to become comfortable with who they are. Books aimed at helping women "rediscover" themselves are selling millions of copies. The website iVillage.com, which touts itself as a home to the authentic woman, is among the most visited site by women on the Internet. Women are being taken seriously as consumers and heads of households. Television networks, like Lifetime and the Oprah Winfrey–backed Oxygen, deliver women-specific entertainment to this powerful group of viewers. Women are finding their voices. It's a very exciting time to be a thirty-one-year-old woman. I am one of those women finding her voice. And I'll tell you . . . once you learn to yell out loud, there's no shutting you up. So what does all of this have to do with running? I'm assuming you bought this book because you have a slight, maybe even semi-serious interest in running. Well, to follow through on the metaphor above, running is a way to exercise the vocal chords. To whisper. To sing. To giggle. And to scream at the top of your lungs.

A few years ago, a woman from work who knew that I ran came up to me and began asking me question after question about running. She had always flirted with the idea of running, but she had many questions and concerns. Plainly put, she didn't know where to start. What kind of shoes to buy, where to go, how far to run. And her biggest question: Do people really enjoy running after all?

In writing this book I talked with women runners across the country, and I discovered that my friend's concerns and curiosities were common ones. Many women like the idea of running, they just don't know if it's for them. Well, that's why I wrote this book. To address those concerns and curiosities, and answer the big question with a resounding *YES*!: Women actually do enjoy running, and you can, too.

In my early twenties, before I started running regularly, I envied those people who were passionate about their health and exercise, especially runners. I always wanted to be one of those women who identified themselves as a "runner." But I never believed it could be me. I didn't believe I would ever enjoy running enough to keep at it for more than a few months. I was wrong. This is not to say I don't have days when the very thought of lacing up my running shoes and walking out the front door is downright exhausting. But I have found a place in my life where running has become integral. And yes, after a few days of no running, I do get a little stir crazy.

What you should know about me as a runner is that while I've been doing it for many years, I'm a runner who continually struggles with motivation. For me, running is a conscious choice I make—harder when my life is particularly hectic, and easier on beautiful fall Sundays that remind me why I started running in the first place. But despite the fact that running is something I have to continually recommit to, I do commit to it. Time and time again. That's probably because I never feel more focused, more healthy and more at peace with myself than after a good run. Running is extremely consistent in its rewards. And so I keep coming back for more.

As you'll discover in this book, I approach running the way I do the rest of my life—rationally. I believe in goal setting, achieving, self-fulfillment and emotional well-being. Running provides me with all of these things. It has enriched my life. I'd even go so far as to say that it has saved it at times. Running has gotten me through some of the lowest moments of my life, and given me an outlet for personal pain. But more important, it's given me an endless source of joy. While I'm not a world-class athlete, I have been running in some capacity for more than fifteen years. I've been trained by elite athletes and coaches, and have learned a lot along the way. While my background is by no means a prerequisite to being a runner, I hope to share what I've learned with you—the potential runner, the beginning runner or even the regular runner in search of more information or motivation.

Inside this book, you'll find information on:

- The physical, emotional, social and mental benefits of running

- How and when to stretch

- Specific concerns for women runners

- How to begin and build your running program

- What to wear

- Where to run

- How to eat to run

- How to stay motivated

- Whether road races are for you

- The importance of cross-training

My ultimate goal in writing this book was to inspire more women to run. What I didn't realize when I began this process was that the incredible people I met along the way and interviewed to supply the quotes throughout this book would inspire me so. Speaking with women I've never met before about how running has impacted their lives led to many long phone conversations and a shared sense of experience that has touched me indescribably. Take the time to read the quotes along the margins as you go through this book, and you'll see what I mean. What I learned most of all, is that running is the ideal sport for women. Its impact is far-reaching to women of all ages, backgrounds and life experiences. If you picked up this book, running is something that you've thought about doing, even if you've never taken the first steps. Well, now you have. Give yourself a gift and read on. You can be a runner, too.

1.

Did You Say Sweat?

Making a Commitment to Being Fit

My mom started exercising for the very first time when she turned forty-eight. For as long as I can remember, my mom's weight has fluctuated, dropping after months of weighing and measuring food as part of her Weight Watchers program (this was before the now popular "points" system), and then creeping back up again to where she started (or beyond) once the diet was "over." But when her doctor told her she was at high risk for diabetes if she didn't take off some weight and lower her blood sugar levels, it was a wake-up call for her. She's been a regular exerciser ever since.

My mom and I talk on the phone a few times a week—with our weekend call being the official "catch-up" call. During one of these long phone conversations, back when she was still in the first few months of exercising, we got to talking about what a huge change it had been to make room in her life for physical fitness after forty-eight years of doing nothing. I suggested that she look at exercising like brushing your teeth—it's something we should do if we want our bodies to stay healthy as we grow older. Who wants to go through life with a chronic toothache, or worse yet, extremely bad breath?

But even though we may intellectually know that exercising is an important component of being a healthy, fit, emotional, productive and fulfilled woman, many of us still haven't made the plunge. How about you? When was the last time you exercised? Went to the gym, went for a jog, took an aerobics class? Earlier today? Yesterday? Last week? Last month? According to the Surgeon General, more than 25 percent of American women don't take part in any sort of physical activity. None. The extent of these women's workouts comes from the occasional stairs in their life, or from any walking they may do in their daily routine. The same Surgeon General report found that many women who do exercise don't do so with the intensity and/or the regularity they need to do to make lasting positive impacts in their lives. And it's women, more often than men, who aren't paying enough attention to exercising. Why do you think that is? I have one theory—that many women take on much more in their lives, physically and emotionally, than many of their male counterparts. We tend to spread ourselves so thin between family and work obligations, that exercise may seem like a luxury to many women. It is, but only in that it's an invaluable gift you give to yourself.

What is Exercise?

So, what does "regular exercise" mean anyway? The definition varies, depending on your sources. The common guidelines for regular exercise are *twenty to thirty minutes of aerobic activity at least three times a week*. This is the *minimum* you should exercise if you want to see some tangible results with regards to your health. And for those twenty to thirty minutes, you should really get the blood pumping through your veins and push your heart so it's getting a workout, too. According to the American Heart Association, a person exercising thirty minutes three to four days a week will achieve cardiovascular fitness, which will help to prevent heart disease, lower blood pressure and improve overall health.

Regular exercise equals twenty to thirty minutes of intense aerobic activity at least three times a week.

There is an easy way you can make sure you're working out hard enough to see some benefits: identify and measure your heart rate before, during and after exercise.

Measuring Your Heart Rate

In case you haven't measured your heart rate before, all you're really doing is checking and noting your pulse. You can do this either on the flat inside of your wrist or along the side of your neck just below the jawbone. There are many different

As I get older, I feel my body changing and I know staying fit is the key to a healthy lifestyle.
Shareena, 32

ways to count and keep track of your heart rate. Make sure you have a clock with a second hand or a digital timer. You can either 1) count the number of beats for a full minute, 2) count the number of beats for fifteen seconds and multiply by four, or 3) count the number of beats for six seconds and add a zero onto the end of your number.

60 seconds = heart rate (eg: 68)

15 seconds × 4 = heart rate (eg: 17 × 4 = 68)

6 seconds and add a zero = heart rate (eg: 7 add zero on end = 70)

All three of these methods will give you a general total that represents your heart rate. If you've got a clock with a second hand nearby, try checking your heart rate right now. The number you come up with should be an approximate representation of your **resting heart rate,** assuming that you're reading this in a comfortable chair or in bed. Once you get used to finding your pulse, checking your heart rate will become second nature.

Target and Maximum Heart Rate (MHR)

I used to smoke and run and I reached a point where I had to make a choice. I loved running so much. So I set a target and I quit smoking. And I went on to reach all my running goals.
Janet, 51

So, how do you make sure you're exercising at the right intensity? The answer is a very individual thing, but now that you know how to measure your heart rate, you will be able to figure it out. You can start by figuring out your personal maximum heart rate or MHR. While your heart rate is a literal representation of the number of heartbeats per minute that your body generates, your maximum heart rate describes the highest number of beats per minute your heart should safely beat. To figure out your personal MHR, there is a simple equation to follow: **226–your age = MHR**. I'm thirty-one years old. So my MHR is 195 beats per minute.

Exercising at our MHR is too intense, and in fact, dangerous. You should aim to have your heart rate at **sixty to eighty percent** of your personal MHR. This is called your **Target Heart Rate.** So, going back to my personal example, if my MHR is 195 beats per minute, then I'd want to make sure my heart rate is at sixty to eighty percent of this amount during exercise. So I take 195 and multiply it by .60 (equals 117) and then multiply 195 by .80 (equals 156). Therefore, my target heart rate is between 117–156 beats per minute. Any higher than 156 beats per minute is too intense for me to sustain safely, and at any less than 117, I would start to lose the health benefits of exercising.

I check my heart rate several times while I'm working out, because I want to make sure that I'm in the zone that I want to be exercising in to get the greatest benefits.
Michele, 33

- **Resting Heart Rate** is your heart rate when not engaging in any exercise.
- **Maximum Heart Rate (MHR)** is the maximum rate your heart should reach. Approximately 226 – your age.
- **Target Heart Rate (THR)** is your goal during exercise. Approximately 60–80 percent of your MHR.

Be aware that while MHR and THR are very individual, the numbers you come up with should be used primarily as indicators, but not absolutes. Differences in heart size and other factors mean that the generally approved guidelines should be taken with a grain of salt. But as you get to know your body and determine your normal resting heart rate, you'll get to know what MHR and THR work for you.

I think exercising does something to the chemicals in your body. Plus you're moving in the right direction toward what you want, and that feels great.
Alice, 34

How It All Fits Together

This isn't to say that you need to check your heart rate at every stage of a workout, nor does this have to be a part of every run. But as you begin your fitness and running program, especially if you're new to exercising in general, it's a good idea to check your heart rate before, during and after your runs. It will help you get to know your body better, and you'll start to get in touch with your heart. You'll probably find that after a while, you'll know instinctively when you're at your ideal aerobic level of activity, because you'll be able to feel it.

Remember, heart rate is a very individual thing. Some people can reach their ideal aerobic level of intensity simply by fast walking. Others may need to really push themselves when they run to maintain their ideal. How fit a person is will determine how intensely they'll need to exercise to get a good aerobic workout. And as you continue to expand on your fitness regimen and make running a bigger part of your life, you may find the same workout that once brought you to your THR isn't intense enough anymore.

If you want to regularly keep track of your heart rate when you exercise, there are digital watches that automatically check your heart rate—no counting, no finding pulse, no nothing. This is an easy way to monitor your heart rate at any stage of your workout, whether you're warming up, walking, running or cooling down.

Women and Exercise

Exercise for the Right Reasons

Are you surprised at the statistics I included earlier about the number of women who aren't exercising? When you think about it, to do the bare minimum in terms of exercise, what we're really talking about is an hour commitment per week. So, why aren't women making exercise a permanent part of their lives?

Here is another theory. It's okay if you disagree. I think one of the biggest reasons why so many women don't exercise regularly is that from the get-go, they choose to exercise for the wrong reasons. The number-one wrong reason I'm talking about is to lose weight. Then when their reasons don't pan out quickly, they quit. I'm certainly not blameless in this category. There have been many times in the past fifteen years when I've vowed to become slender, and exercised like a madwoman on a mission. The first problem here is that my body has no intention of *ever* being slender. I'm a muscular gal. If anything, I tend to gain weight when I exercise frequently. Yet, even knowing this, I have repeatedly launched into a heavy exercise regimen with a mental image of a lean, toned, svelte woman in my head, expecting some sort of a metamorphosis on my butt and thighs. And with unrealistic goals like this, I am bound to be disappointed. And so are many other women who are on similar missions.

So what happens? When the primary motivation is gone, workouts are skipped, and hence, exercise plans fail. My sister recently drove this point home with me. Last month, she called and left a message on my voicemail at work, saying, "Call me.

I've become tremendously more confident about what I can do physically than I was before. I'm not a fast runner, but I just think of myself as a more athletic person, which gives me more confidence. I really like having that. Sarah, 28

It's urgent. Page me if you have to." My sister's emergency amounted to her discouragement at not losing a single pound in her first few weeks of working out and eating well, despite the pretty radical change she was making in her routine. "Should I keep going?" she asked me. "Will I eventually see results?" she desperately asked. What could I say, but "Yes! Of course! Keep going!" I didn't guarantee her that she'd lose weight if she continued on her eating and exercising streak, although I believed she would. Instead, I took the "what's the worst that can happen" approach. I assured her that exercising could only positively impact her in so many ways, and that not exercising was, well, *not exercising*. By not working out and eating poorly, my sister could pretty much guarantee that nothing was going to change with regards to her weight and health. In fact, experts now say that a sedentary lifestyle is as bad for you as a smoking lifestyle!

> *For me, real exercise is aerobic, and in my mind I think that if I do anything less than thirty minutes, it's not enough.*
> *Bridget, 32*

Many exercise programs fail because participants start them for the wrong reasons. To make exercise a true part of your life, dig below the surface and set goals that are attainable and good for the soul.

What about you? Are you reading this now and thinking that you, too, imagine a sleek, muscular you, clad in running shorts, tanned and looking awesome? I can't guarantee that running will transform your body into the picture you have in your head. But, I can say without doubt that if you make a commitment to fitness you will feel better about yourself and your body. Just knowing that you're doing something so good for yourself is pretty wonderful. I'm sure many of you have experienced a "high" of sorts after a good workout. Well, when you're exercising regularly, a little bit of that high always stays with you. You'll think about yourself differently, more positively. And your reflection in the mirror will be more forgiving with the knowledge that you're taking steps to nurture yourself.

I used to take body sculpting aerobic classes with an instructor named Kendall. She was tall, extremely fit, with long, well-defined muscles, and was one of the most motivational instructors I had ever had. About two years after I stopped taking her class, I read an article in a local magazine about personal trainers who used plastic surgery, including liposuction, to achieve their physical appearance. Kendall was one of the trainers portrayed in the article as having had liposuction twice. I can't tell you how bummed out I was to read that. I even felt a little betrayed.

Unfortunately, self-image is really at the heart of the matter for most of us. We are obsessed with our bodies—our thighs, our butts, our hips, our stomachs. My own obsession has always been my thighs, which have been strong and muscular (read "large") from an early age because of my training as a gymnast. That and genetics. For as long as I can remember, I have yearned for long, slender legs. And a few years ago it finally sunk in. I'm never going to have long, slender legs. My calves will always be large. My ankles thick. My thighs? Forget about it. They will always remain . . . shapely.

For many of us, this obsession and dissatisfaction with our bodies can be all consuming. Ask around. How many women do you know who are happy with their bodies? How many women look in the mirror in their undies and say, "Damn, I look good!" More likely, they're standing in front of the mirror doing the pencil/butt test. (For those of you who aren't familiar

Exercise provides me with self-awareness, and it feels healthy. Therefore, it's exhilarating to me.
Gail, 52

I think about staying in shape as I get older, to be healthy and to be happy with the way I look.
Christie, 29

with this, it involves a pencil and your butt, and draws attention to the possibility of your being able to hold a pencil in the fleshy area between the bottom of your butt and the back of your thigh. If the pencil stays in place, then the test dictates there's too much "sagging" going on back there. My recommendation—avoid doing this test!) The worst part about this is when we are feeling down or insecure about our bodies, it creeps into our psyche and affects how we value ourselves, and ultimately how others perceive us. It is a vicious cycle, and one that we need to break.

I think the image of the ideal woman used to be worse. At least recently a more athletic and capable orientation has come into that image. But whatever that image is, it's unattainable.
Libby, 41

Something bigger has to change. Our attitudes (and society's attitudes) about what is and isn't sexy, attractive and alluring need to be adjusted. This is no easy task, especially considering the messages being drilled into us by the media—that we as women need to be supermodel skinny to be happy, find a partner, and secure everything that is good in this world. I remember one particularly annoying ad campaign for Kellogg's Special K cereal. You know, the one with a commercial that features a bony, hipless woman drooling over her own reflection as she squeezes into a size two dress, *oohing* and *aahing* all the way? I was happy to discover Kellogg's dropped that campaign several years ago, after women consumers complained the ads portrayed "an unrealistically thin and unhealthy body image as the ideal."

And after all, health is what we're after here. Kudos to Kellogg's for developing a new campaign aimed at promoting positive self-images for women. It's a start. Unfortunately, all too many women continue to ignore their better senses, and their genetic makeup for that matter, by trying every diet in the book in an attempt to look like the very model described above. You name it, I've tried it at some point: Eat to Win, the Zone, Weight Watchers, even that strange diet that had women across the country making vats of celery and cabbage soup. The reality is, while these diets may result in immediate weight loss, and sometimes even substantial poundage, the losses are invariably short-term. Just like my mom, dieters all too often find themselves right back where they started after their body figures out what's going on. This is not to say that some diets and eating plans can't be beneficial, but they need to be about life change, not short-term benefits. Yet each and every month, one out of every three women is on one diet or another.

What I suggest is a more permanent change. A win-win situation. And here's what I mean. If I am running regularly, then logic dictates that my legs and thighs cannot be "fat." It's just plain common sense. If I am running regularly, logic dictates that I can't be unhealthy and out of shape. Again, that common sense thing. This might seem like a moot argument, but I still use it when I'm bloated during PMS and feeling very bad about my body. Sometimes, this common sense is what I rely on the most to get me through a run. While running regularly may not give you a supermodel's legs, or a triathlete's build, it can certainly give your legs tone and positively change their shape by reducing your body's overall body fat and increasing the percentage of muscle. As I said before, I have come to accept that my thighs will always be "shapely." And that is what they're des-

Exercise has toughened me up. I don't mean just physically, I mean mentally. It's hard for me to think there's something out there that I can't confront.
Paulette, 50

tined to be. But I guarantee you this. If you begin a regular exercise program, stick to it, and make it a part of your life, you will become healthy. You will keep your weight at a good range for you and your body type. You will feel good about yourself. And you'll learn to accept your body—thighs, butt and all—for what they are. Yours.

The Greatness of Exercising Regularly

While looking and feeling good is undoubtedly a goal in any exercise program, just as important is the notion of achieving "wellness"—a state of physical fitness and wellness wherein your body works more effectively. It's no secret that the higher your level of overall health and wellness, the better able your body is to fight against sickness, turn food into energy more efficiently, keep you mentally healthy. When you're exercising, everything in your body just seems to work better.

Women who frequently exercise have overall increased energy, increased life expectancy, and lower levels of stress and tension. Women exercisers tend to sleep better, think clearer when they're awake, and have more emotional stability than their nonexercising counterparts. According to a 1991 Harvard Graduate School of Public

SOME BENEFITS OF EXERCISING . . .

- Sleep better
- Think clearer
- Live longer
- Feel less stressful
- Be more emotionally stable
- Have better overall health

Health study conducted by Dr. Rose Frisch, "Young women who participated in college sports or exercised regularly during college were significantly less likely to contract breast cancer." And it's a known fact that women and girls who participate in sports do better academically, and later down the road, professionally. As moms, women can be positive role models for their daughters and get them involved in exercise early on in their lives—the rewards they'll experience later in life will be great.

Make a Commitment and Set Goals

So. What do you say? Are you willing to give it a go? I'll say this one more time. You have absolutely NOTHING TO LOSE and EVERYTHING TO GAIN. As you move forward in committing to an exercise regimen, start to think about a goal or two that you can set at this stage. Nothing too fancy or aggressive. Maybe it's just a simple goal to get you to the next chapter, and one page closer to lacing up your running shoes and going out for a jog. Keep it realistic. In other words, a goal of completing a triathlon or dropping twenty pounds in the next month might not be a safe bet. Be nice to yourself. Set some goals that you can achieve and feel good about. There's nothing like achieving a goal to keep you moving forward.

Here are some suggested goals as you embark on your exercise program. Use one of these, or come up with one of your own!

I exercise to have some peace of mind, time alone to let my train of thought go where it might, and to have more energy in the long run.
Dayla, 26

- Finish reading this book

- Exercise "regularly" for one month (at least three times per week, 20 minutes each time)

- Start an exercise journal

- Write down the steps you will take to make exercise a true part of your life

---

I commit to make exercise a part of my life. I know that exercising and nurturing my body is an expression of self-love—a way of celebrating my spiritual and physical being. As part of my commitment to a healthier lifestyle, I set the goal of:

_____

_____

_____

_____

Signed _____

Dated _____

2.

Why Become a Runner?

The (Many) Benefits of Running

How do I love running? Let me count the ways. I run for many different reasons, depending on where I "am" in my life, both emotionally and physically. During my college years and when I first moved to New York City, running was the only form of exercise I could afford. After shelling out the money for a pair of running shoes, I was ready to go, be it on the sidewalks, the roads, or in Central Park. Running has been like a friend to me since I was in middle school. It's something I can always count on. Sometimes I focus on things as simple as the sound of leaves crackling under my feet, the feeling of the sun beating down on my bare shoulders or the smell of freshly cut grass. Other times I tune into my body and focus within. It always brings me pleasure and boosts my self-confidence a few notches, no matter how low it sinks. And no one can take running away from me. And that has always empowered me.

I know that for many women, the very thought of running is

absolutely painful. I know this because I have friends who respond in amazement when I tell them I'm a runner, quizzically asking, "How can you do that? It just hurts so much." Even watching others run can drum up visions of aches and pains in some women. I believe a lot of that anxiety comes from the unknown. Running on some level has been mystified, as if runners are a special secret society, and only a very few people have access to the password that actually makes it a pleasant experience. Not true. Really. It's just not true. So, before we get ahead of ourselves, maybe it's best to first talk about all of the WONDERFUL things about running. And there are lots of them.

Physical Benefits of Running

Many women probably begin a running program with a physical goal foremost in their minds, like losing some weight or toning their legs. These are definitely some potential physical benefits of running, but they're not the only ones. There are many different physical side effects of running that will make a difference in any woman's life.

RUNNING CAN (AND WILL) . . .

- Tone your legs
- Increase your bone mass
- Lower cholesterol
- Lower blood pressure
- Strengthen your heart
- Reduce risk of breast cancer
- Boost your immune system
- Clear your complexion
- Speed up recovery time from injury and sickness
- Control your weight
- Improve your sex life

Improvement of Overall Health

One of the greatest benefits of a running lifestyle is that it strongly contributes to a woman's overall health in so many ways. While much national attention is given to the epidemic of heart disease in men, heart disease is also the number-one cause of death for women in the U.S. Running and other cardiovascular activities are excellent ways to strengthen the heart and ensure the efficient flow of blood and oxygen throughout the body—things that are proven to help to decrease the risk of heart attack.

I used to get sick so much more often before I was running, and I don't get sick anymore. I know that running has boosted my immune system. Christie, 29

One of the first things a doctor will tell you if you have hypertension, or high blood pressure, is to start exercising. Exercise, combined with maintaining a healthy weight, is one of the best ways to naturally reduce your blood pressure if it's above normal. I happen to have high blood pressure—I have for years (thanks, Mom!). Running and eating a low sodium diet has kept it in check for the most part. Another thing running has helped me control is my once-high cholesterol (thanks, Dad!). I'm happy to say that my running, along with eating relatively healthily, has naturally lowered my cholesterol. In fact, at my last doctor's appointment, my cholesterol level actually placed me in a normal to better-than-average group.

And the more miles you run, the more health benefits you'll reap. According to a National Runner's Health Study, "The benefits of running forty miles per week versus under ten miles can be dramatic. Women in the forty-mile club reduce their risk of cardiovascular disease by an estimated 45 percent." Now, forty miles a week is a lot. Right now I'm averaging about twenty-five to thirty, and that's pretty high for me. But it is good to know that we can have a certain degree of control over our physical being and our health as we continue to age. And that the more effort we put in, the more rewards we'll reap.

Some of the other overall beneficial side effects of running and other cardiovascular exercise include:

• **More efficient immune system**—Your body functions more efficiently and is better able to fend off those nasty germs, so you'll have a better chance of avoiding that cold that's circulating around the office.

• **Arthritis control**—According to the Surgeon General, running and other cardiovascular exercise can actually help control the joint swelling and pain that goes along with arthritis.

• **Breast cancer prevention**—According to the Journal of the National Cancer Institute, "One to three hours of exercise a week over a woman's reproductive lifetime [the teens to about age 40] may bring a 20 percent to 30 percent reduction in the risk of breast cancer, and four or more hours of exercise a week can reduce the risk almost 60 percent." Those are odds I'd like to take.

• **Increased bone density**—As women, we're susceptible to suffering from osteoporosis (a decrease in our bone density due to loss of calcium) as we age. Running, and other weight-bearing exercises, increases bone density, which can fend off osteoporosis.

• **Healthier skin**—Running improves circulation, which in turn encourages your body to flush out waste products and fat deposits that can affect your skin and complexion.

Prevention of and Quicker Recovery from Injury

In the spring of 1996, I broke my ankle playing tennis. It was an especially harsh blow because I was just starting to run more regularly after coming out of my winter "hibernation," and had signed up for a whole bunch of road races. I was in a cast for six weeks—on crutches for half of that time, and in a walking cast for the other half. By the time my cast came off that July, my left leg from the knee down was a shriveled (and hairy) muscleless stick. My quadricep wasn't in much better condition. My orthopedist said that I could expect the process of reversing the atrophy (decrease in muscle size from inactivity) in my leg to last upwards of a year. Discouraged to say the least, I started working out again, first through aerobics, then walking, and eventually running. Within two months my left leg was about equal in size to the right one. I even went on to run my first marathon that November. I know that if I hadn't been in good shape with strong leg muscles prior to that fated tennis game, my recovery process would have been much more lengthy.

It's a known fact that the better physical shape you're in the quicker you'll recover from any injuries. But being in good shape can help you prevent getting injured in the first place. Many of us hurt ourselves by almost silly accidents—tripping over a crack in the sidewalk, stepping incorrectly off of a curb. The better shape you're in, the more quickly and efficiently your muscles and

After being sickly with asthma for so long when I was little, running was something I never thought I could do. Now that I can, it feels so cool.
Alice, 34

I started to run in college when everyone's worried about gaining the "freshman fifteen." Running helped me to gain a new self-confidence and not worry about all of that.

Emily, 29

reflexes are able to react in these kinds of situations, and the less likely you are to hurt yourself in the first place.

Weight Control

While I know I went on and on in the last chapter about immediate weight loss being the wrong motivation for an exercise program, there is no denying that weight control is a positive side effect of running. Any form of aerobic or cardiovascular activity results in the burning of calories. Consequently, burning more calories than you are eating will eventually result in some weight loss. Running is near the top of the list of activities that burn the most calories per minute (approximately one hundred calories per mile), along with fast walking and swimming. The chart below represents calories burned per minute of running and jogging:

ACTIVITY	105–115 LBS	127–137 LBS	160–170 LBS	182–192 LBS
Jogging (12-minute miles)	8.6	9.8	11.5	12.7
Running ($\frac{7}{12}$-minutes miles)	10.4	11.9	14.1	15.5

From Your Health, 1990, Prentice Hall

Likewise, running and other cardiovascular exercise also speeds up your metabolism and keeps it running faster even after you've finished your workout, so you'll burn more calories in everything you do. For me, running has been more of a form of maintaining a normal, healthy weight rather than as a tool for quick weight loss. One thing to keep in mind about running is that the more you run, the more you will need to eat to fuel your body. As I'm now training for a marathon, which includes one long run per week, I have to make sure I'm eating enough "energy" foods to give me the fuel I need to finish my runs. While training for this marathon, I've actually gained about five pounds—probably a combination of increased muscle mass and well, just eating more food.

I started running in 1977 when I was in grad school, because I had gained weight over the winter. I was in Michigan, so we had cold winters, and we had all kinds of good things to eat. Paulette, 50

Everyone's metabolism is different. Generally speaking, a woman's metabolism tends to be slower than a man's. And it's also thought that every five years or so our metabolism gets slower. So we'll need to increase our workouts to yield the same results. As I mentioned, I've been gaining weight while training for this marathon, while I've actually lost weight while training for marathons in the past. It's a fact that runners' bodies react differently to distance training—some gain weight, others lose weight. Some stay the same. I'm sure that part of my personal weight gain is attributable to an increase in muscle, which weighs more than fat. But regardless, I know that as long as I keep running as a part of my lifestyle, and continue to eat relatively healthily with only occasional indulgences of Krispy Kreme donuts and other such delights, I'm going to keep my weight at a place that is healthy and not put a strain on my heart.

Improved Sex Life

You'll have to judge this one for yourself (and with your partner, of course). According to sex therapist Linda De Villers, Ph.D., women between the ages of 18 and 45 who exercise three times a week reported the following results about their own sex lives:

- 25 percent reported feeling more "frisky" after a workout
- 40 percent reported feeling more sexually responsive
- 31 percent reported having sex more often
- 25 percent reported having orgasms more frequently
- 80 percent reported having more sexual confidence

I'll spare you the details of my own personal sex life, but I will say that I feel much more attractive and good about myself and my body when I'm running. And I never feel more attractive than after a long, hard run (after showering, of course).

Emotional and Mental Benefits of Running

So, enough about all the physical benefits. If I were to tell you what I love *best* about running, it's *the way running makes me feel.* Hands down. And women *feel* a lot of things. It's part of what makes us so wonderful—our ability to feel things deeply. Granted, some of us are more emotional than others in how we express our feelings. I'm one of those tipping the scale in the "expressing emotions" department. In fact, when my husband, Derin, and I first started dating, I used to be embarrassed about my emotional nature. I was surprised to find that he liked my emotional side—to him it represented my capacity to experience life. And for all of the times I'm down emotionally or feeling pain because of a situation, the highs are all

Running is the best thing in the world when it's over. Not because it's done, but more just the way you feel. Once you get over that hump of when you think you're going to die and then you keep going, it's great.
Amy, 30

that much better. Running and the way it makes me feel has played a huge part in defining who I am—how I perceive myself, how I handle problems, how I process information.

The Wonder of Endorphins

I'm sure you've heard of the phrase "runner's high," which describes a euphoric feeling that some runners experience during or after a run. Well, there's actually a physiological cause for this "high"—endorphins. *Endorphins* literally means "morphine within" and this literal translation should give you an indication of what they do in your body. Endorphins are actually painkilling proteins in the brain, and strenuous exercises like running can release them into the bloodstream, resulting in the runner experiencing a positive, euphoric-like feeling. Ask several runners what they love best about running, and at least one will say it's the way they feel afterwards. This is a result of endorphins moving through the bloodstream, making the runner feel mentally clear and refreshed. In endorphins we have a natural painkiller, with no negative side effects!

Self-Esteem and Self-Image

I think we could all use a little help in the self-esteem department. And unfortunately, young girls are struggling with self-image crises earlier and earlier in life. And these issues carry over into adulthood. As I mentioned earlier, I have been active in sports for most of my life—first gymnastics and then track. I never gave a second thought to my body and my weight in my

When I graduated from college, I was an insomniac, and I would run at one A.M. or two A.M. because I couldn't do anything else. It became this really amazing time by myself, meditative and everything like that.
Maggie, 25

younger years, except for that big question: *When in the world was I going to grow breasts?* (Not until the eleventh grade, it turned out!) But beyond that, I was just fine with my weight, my butt, my thighs and my calves. Until spring track my junior year in high school. I remember the first time I put on my track outfit, consisting of standard eighties fare—short blue silky running shorts and a matching tank top. One of my male coaches looked at me and asked me what happened to me over the last year, indicating that I looked a lot bigger than I had in the past. If I was smart, I would have replied, "It's called puberty. Duh." But I didn't. Instead I went home and weighed myself, confirming that I was about ten pounds heavier than the year before. And so began my days (and my life) of being self-conscious and critical of my body. I'm sure each woman reading this can pinpoint that moment when she first became aware of her own body and held it up against the ridiculous image of the "ideal" that the media portrays. It's not a pretty day. Unless you're one of the .01 percent of the population that actually fits this description.

I love the way running makes me feel physically, emotionally and mentally. It makes me feel like an athlete, and nothing's ever done that before.
Christie, 29

Low self-esteem can be paralyzing. We're not in control of the images that the media throws around on the cover of women's magazines. And most of us will never look like those images; (again, .01 percent excluded). So taking control of our self-image and building our self-esteem are very powerful actions. It's no joke that women who feel better about themselves are perceived as more attractive. Attitude can go a long way. And I guarantee you that making running a part of your life will boost your self-esteem and make you feel better about yourself and your body. There are so many things that contribute to this boost in self-esteem. There's the challenge of setting a goal for yourself and working to accomplish it. That very act is so empowering, and it gives us back some control in our otherwise hectic and crazy lives. There's the very act of running itself; it may not always feel wonderful, but you're out there doing it. You're running while others are just walking. Or sitting around. I mean, come on—you're out there running, for goodness sake. You're to be taken seriously! And then, there's the way you feel after a run—my favorite part. It's an exhaustion like no other. Things shift into focus. Priorities become clear. And that bit of cellulite along the back of your thigh isn't quite so significant when you've been out there running, sweating, working and breathing.

For me, running is a worship experience. I feel like it's bringing myself centered—emotionally, physically, mentally. I love nature, too, so I enjoy all those senses of seeing, smelling and sweating. It's a total body experience. Karen, 39

Running helps us take control of our self-image and recreate our own sense of beauty.

There is no limit to the emotional rewards you can reap from running. That's because there are always new goals to set and new challenges to meet. And every time you surpass a goal you didn't think was possible, your self-esteem and confidence sky-rocket. All of my life I had wanted to run a marathon. But I was (and still am) a sprinter. Frankly, my body just isn't built for endurance or long distance. As of five years ago, the most I had ever run was six or seven miles. But it was one of those things I always wanted to do, just to accomplish it. I may not have ever run that first marathon in 1996 if a colleague hadn't been on the committee for the New York Marathon and asked me with only two months notice if I wanted to run. Faced with the real opportunity I hesitantly said yes. Two months later when I crossed the finish line in just under five hours, I cried in a swell of emotion. It just came out of me. I had done something I believed I couldn't do. To me, the marathon was the ultimate

SOME GREAT EMOTIONAL SIDE EFFECTS OF RUNNING:

- **Empowerment**
- **Achievement**
- **Accomplishment**
- **Satisfaction**
- **Contentment**

I had never gotten into a fitness routine that worked for me, but running was a fit. When I ran my first mile and I realized I could do it, that's all it took. That was five years ago.
AnneMarie, 32

When I wake up in the morning, I can't wait to get my shoes on and go for a run. I just feel it's the best part of my day.
Janet, 51

personal challenge. It was something I had built up in my head to be a sacred event. That marathon affected me for months after it was over. I felt so good about myself, so proud of myself and so unstoppable. It was like a year's worth of therapy rolled into one Sunday afternoon.

Self-esteem is a cumulative commodity. You don't gain some and then have it fritter away again. With each day of running, and each challenge faced, your self-esteem will just grow and grow. Feeling good about yourself can become second nature. And making running a part of your life can speed up that process for you.

Mental Toughness

The notion of mental toughness is tied to my marathon experience, but it's a significant side effect of running and deserves separate mention. I wrote earlier that a lot of women ask me how I can stand to run when it just hurts so much. And there is something to be said about the fact that running doesn't always feel like flannel pajamas under a down comforter on a cool spring morning. But to some degree, it's overcoming the physical challenges of running that make it so rewarding.

I have been running road races for about seven years now. And no matter how many I run, I have yet to run one where I don't think about stopping, dropping out, or walking at least once. I would have thought that it would eventually start to get easier. That running races would become this kind of routine event, and that once I had experienced the physical discomfort of pushing my body and muscles to the limit, it wouldn't really faze me too much anymore. Wrong. It fazes me. A lot. It's part of the internal discussion I have with myself during each race, challenging myself to make it to the next water stop or mile marker. But when I do persevere and I make it through the whole race, pushing through the pain and even allowing myself to experience it to some degree, the feeling of accomplishment at the end is all that much more intense.

If you have a chance to watch a road race, check out the faces of the women near the front of the pack—the women who are really pushing themselves. They look tough. They look focused. They look like they've got a job to do and every ounce of will and energy in their body is working together to get it done. Now think about applying that same degree of mental toughness to difficult situations in life that we all face. We are so capable of dealing with and even thriving against the most adverse of circumstances, but we don't have a lot of experience testing our abilities. You don't have to be a top runner to appreciate the effects of mental toughness. Go for a run in the rain. Cold rain. When it starts to rain harder, tag another five minutes onto your run instead of cutting it short. You'll finish that run more mentally tough than when you began it. And just like self-esteem, mental toughness continues to grow

> I feel like a self-sufficient machine when I run. It wakes up all of my organs and brings me to life. It can hurt, but when you work through the pain, you feel that much stronger.
> Laurie, 31

> I used to drink too much, and I got sober. But my mind was going too fast. If I could get my mind and body going at the same speed, then everything was fine. My sponsor would say, "Maggie, when's the last time you ran?" and she'd tell me to go for a run. And inevitably it would help.
> Maggie, 25

Running and PMS: running while experiencing PMS or during your period helps alleviate the pain that accompanies these times. The endorphins that running releases in your body are natural pain relievers!

with every run you do. And you'll be much better prepared to handle any of those curves life throws at you as a result.

Quality Personal Time and Clarity

I feel like a couples' therapist when I talk about "quality time." Or I think back to my father who wouldn't let us watch TV during dinner, because that was our "quality family time." Well, running can offer you some of the best quality personal time there is.

Running makes me feel like I have superpowers. I used to dream that I was running and I'd wake up and think "I'll never be able to do that." Now that I can, it's truly a superpower! Michele, 33

This is perhaps one of my personal favorite benefits of running. Running is my time to process. To analyze. Or to zone out. I'll solve problems, brainstorm or plan the rest of my day. Some of my favorite runs are those when I'm so busy thinking about something that the run becomes incidental. Years ago when I was in between jobs, a former boss called to see if I'd go to Rwanda for a film shoot about the crisis happening there. I left my temp job, my head flooded with ideas and excitement and possibility. I ran for an hour that night and by the time I got home from the park I had no recollection of the actual physical run itself. My mind was the only thing I remember racing that night. Thank goodness I was able to run, or I would have spazzed out for days. The run also gave me the time to digest the idea of putting myself in a potentially dangerous environment, and get some clarity on the situation. As it turned out, the trip never happened. But my run that night is still a vivid memory.

If you're running with a partner or a group of people, you'll still have the opportunity to experience this sense of clarity. Depending on your moods, you and your running partner might go through the whole run and not even talk. Derin and I pretty regularly go through runs where we'll both sink into our own little worlds. And then if we want to bounce an idea we've just been thinking about off of each other, we have that option.

There are very few things that get me up at 5:30 in the morning, but running does. It gives me energy.
Colleen, 26

Social Benefits

Runners are pretty great people. And I'm not just saying that because I am one. I've found it to be generally true. I'm not sure what it is about the sport that makes it so, but as a community, runners are friendly, kind and supportive. Not a bad bunch to throw yourself into.

As I look back at the different phases of my life, going back to about sixth grade, my circle of friends has always involved at least a handful of runners. In middle school and high school, my best friends were on the track team. My closest friend from Penn State was someone I ran track with freshman year. In New York, I ran with a group from the United Nations (I worked for UNICEF for years), and had a pretty interesting multinational group of friends to hang out with as a result. And now that we've moved to California, our closest friends are people we run with on a regular basis.

You have an instant camaraderie with anyone who runs. They want to know how much you train, they want to hear your race stories. People love to talk about running.
Janet, 51

Getting involved in running, and more specifically a running organization, is a great way to meet people and make new friends. Most cities have running clubs—the Road Runners' Club of America has more than 600 clubs in forty-eight states across the country alone. And most running clubs have membership activities like group runs, races, social events, fundraisers and running classes. And like I said, runners are nice people!

Running has exposed me to a lot of great people I wouldn't have met otherwise. Sharing race experiences and long weekend runs with a group magnifies the experience for me.
Eileen, 26

I love running with one other person, and I really enjoy running with another woman. I find that it completely takes my mind off of running and I can run so much farther.

Bridget, 32

Running with the UN Track Club was great fun. The weekly group workouts on Wednesday nights were awesome. We'd bundle up in our winter running gear, including hats, gloves and scarves, and we'd weave our way through the streets in the cold dark night to the outdoor track along the East River at Twelfth Street in Manhattan. Then our coach, Jorge, would break us into groups and give us our workouts. When we were done, we'd make our way back to the office, sometimes going out for pizza together after we'd changed back into our warm street clothes. I have fond memories of those nights and the feeling of being a part of a diverse group of people who really didn't have anything in common other than their love of running.

Running Is for Everyone, Anytime, Anywhere

Running really is for just about anyone, and you can do it anytime, just about anywhere. I like to think of running as one of the great equalizers. With very minimal expense—literally the cost of some running shoes—you can have access to the best gym in the world. The world itself. There are many sports that just aren't accessible to everyone. Racquetball, swimming, tennis, golf—all of these cost money for court time, gym time, equipment. But there's no monthly fee to hit the park three times a week for a jog.

Running is one of the only baby-friendly sports—baby buggies are readily available to women who want to share their run with their babies. Talk about a good workout!

You don't have to worry about waiting to get on any equipment or calling ahead to book a court. Running shoes don't discriminate, so women of all ages, backgrounds and ethnic groups can feel free to run without fear. We all grew up running—playing tag or kick the can, chasing after our sisters. It's part of what our body naturally wants to do.

Running is so cheap. It has a huge payoff, with very little up-front investment. Colleen, 26

And the great thing about running is that you can do it just about anywhere. Unless you live in Venice and travel by gondola, there are few places in the world where you can't go for a jog. Whether you're at the beach, in a national park, in a city, or in the desert, there's always a new course to be found. *Have running shoes, will travel!* One note of caution: Be aware that as women we have to take extra precautions when running alone. Make sure that your route is a safe one, and isn't isolated. Run smart.

I want to be one of those people who they announce coming in at a race . . . "Here she comes, our oldest runner, 92-year-old Paulette . . ." Paulette, 50

Running is custom-built for women. And I have yet to meet a woman runner who hasn't experienced at least some of the benefits outlined in this chapter, even in as little as a few weeks of beginning their program. Running is more than a form of exercise—it's a lifestyle. Take the leap and make it a part of yours!

3

What to Wear:

Finding the Right Running Gear

A few years ago, a woman I used to work with was excited because she was just getting into running. So she decided to get a good pair of shoes and went to a sporting goods store one weekend to buy her very first pair of running shoes. The salesman who helped her began by asking how many miles she ran per week, so he could suggest an appropriate pair of shoes. When she replied, "three to five miles," the salesman laughed and suggested perhaps she just buy regular sneakers. My friend left the store embarrassed and discouraged, and without buying any running shoes at all. If that's customer service, who needs it! Venturing into a running or sports store to buy your first pair of running shoes can be an intimidating thing, to say the least. But, the truth is, any woman who plans to run, no matter how many miles, should be fitted with proper running shoes, and should be dressed appropriately for reasons of health, safety and comfort.

Finding the Right Running Shoe

So, while buying the right pair of running shoes can be intimidating, it doesn't have to be. The more informed you are, the better. So, here is some information that will help you figure out what kind of shoe will work best for you before you even get to the store.

Shoes to Match Your Feet and Stride

There are three primary kinds of running shoes: cushioned, stability, and motion control. Which kind of shoe you wear depends on what your feet are like and how you run. Most people fall into one of the following categories: overpronaters, underpronaters, or normal.

My first pair of running shoes was expensive, but I decided that running was my fitness routine. Some people join a gym, some people buy bikes. This was the equipment I needed to do my thing.
AnneMarie, 32

- **Overpronation**—Overpronation is the rolling inward of the feet and ankles when running, or when walking for that matter. Many people who overpronate have relatively flat feet.

- **Underpronation**—Underpronation is the opposite of overpronation—the feet roll excessively to the outside when walking or running. People who underpronate tend to have very high arches.

- **Normal**—People who don't overpronate or underpronate would be considered to have a normal running or walking stride.

One of the easiest ways to figure out if you overpronate or underpronate is to stand without socks on, and pull your pants up to midcalf. Have a friend look (or use a mirror to look yourself) at the back of your legs, from below your calf to the bottom of the heel. If you don't overpronate or underpronate, your ankle bone and the Achilles tendon along the back of your leg will be relatively straight up and down, making a straight line perpendicular to the ground at a ninety degree angle. If you have an overpronation, you or your friend will notice that the insides of your ankles lean slightly inward. If you underpronate, your ankles will lean outward. You can also tell if you over- or underpronate by looking at your wet footprint and getting a sense of how high or low your arches are. If you have high arches, you'll see very little of the middle section of your foot on the footprint (a sign of underpronation). If your footprint shows much or all of the middle section of your foot, this is a sign of flat-footedness (and overpronation). Normal lies somewhere in between these two extremes. Overpronation and underpronation are things that many sports and fitness store employees are trained to recognize. If you're unsure about whether or not you do any of these things, make sure to ask the salesperson where you buy your running shoes.

I tend to underpronate, and I select my running shoes the way I do bathing suits and jeans. Once I find a shoe that works for me, I buy it in every version they come out with.
Colleen, 26

You'll want to be aware of how you run and walk when buying running shoes, because the way your feet land will determine the type of shoe for you.

Cushioned Shoes

Cushioned shoes are designed for people who have either normal stride and feet or for those who underpronate. Because they don't need any extra support in their shoe to keep their heel in place, these runners can buy shoes that focus more on a cushioned run. This doesn't mean that cushioned shoes aren't supportive—they are. But they don't offer the same type of support that you'd find in stability or motion control shoes. The goal of cushioned shoes is to provide a running experience with as much shock absorption in the shoe as possible. This is especially important for heavier runners, as it lessens the impact the rest of your body will have to absorb with each step. Cushioned shoes are generally lightweight compared with other types of shoes.

Motion Control

Motion control shoes have a lot of extra support built into the heel of the shoe, and this severely limits the motion your ankle can make from side to side. These are the best alternative for those who overpronate or have flat feet. The idea is that your heel will remain relatively stable in the shoe. While these shoes have a good degree of cushion, the focus is on a hardier, sturdier shoe. These will usually be substantially heavier than cushioned shoes and stability shoes.

I always run in a good pair of shoes. Right now I'm running in New Balance, because they're a little wider. Deena, 32

Stability

Stability shoes fall somewhere right in the middle between cushioned and motion control shoes. They provide a good deal of support throughout the shoe and particularly the heel area, while still being relatively light and cushiony. I run in stability shoes, although I have a slight overpronation. I used to run in motion control shoes, and started having pain in my heel area, which I attributed to the fact that the shoe was holding my heel too rigidly. I switched to stability shoes about five years ago and I've never looked back. Stability shoes are probably the most common type of running shoes available, as runners with only slight overpronations or underpronations can be served well wearing them.

Trail Shoes

Trail shoes are designed specifically for running crosscountry or on nonpavement like . . . well, like trails. They tend to be a heavier shoe with a fair amount of support to help protect your feet and ankles on rougher terrain. They generally have a pretty substantial tread on the bottom, again, to allow for easier negotiation on surfaces like dirt, rocks, leaves, and so on. While these trail shoes are very hip in design, because they are generally heavier than traditional running shoes, I would advise against making them your everyday running shoe and reserve them for where they do best—the trail.

Racing Shoes

If you do find yourself racing and you want to wear a shoe specifically geared for speed, several shoemakers produce racing shoes, or *racing flats* as they're sometimes called. The key design element in these shoes is that they're very light and simple. They are basically all cushion and not a lot of support. The goal is to keep you as light on your feet as possible, while providing a comfortable ride. But like trail shoes, I would recommend wearing these shoes only in circumstances of running a road race. They're not designed for regular wear and longer distances.

FOOT TYPE	SHOE TYPE
Normal	Stability
Severe overpronation	Motion Control
Moderate to slight overpronation	Motion Control/Stability
Severe underpronation	Cushioned
Moderate to slight underpronation	Cushioned/Stability

How Much Money Should You Spend on Shoes?

Running shoes can range in price from $30 to $150. For example, the Nike Air Max, a very popular running shoe, will run you about $135.00 a pair, while New Balance's top-of-the-line running shoe is about $109.00. Don't feel the need to spend this much money on your shoes. The top-of-the-line shoes are built for runners who log a lot of weekly miles. There are many great running shoes from Adidas, Asics, New Balance and Saucony in the $50–$70 range. So how do you determine which shoe is for you?

I saved my Sauconys from my first marathon and I will never get rid of those shoes. I'd have them bronzed but they're too big.
Janet, 51

Ultimately, running shoes are a very personal thing. I've run in Asics and Sauconys with some regularity, and they both provide different but comfortable running experiences for me. New Balance shoes, on the other hand, are a little too narrow for me. If you have a specialty runners' shop near you, you'll undoubtedly get the best service there and a salesperson can help you make your choice based on the shape of your foot, whether or not you pronate, how frequently you plan to run, and so on. At the Super Runners Shop in New York, all of the employees are runners themselves, and are trained in the specifics of all shoes. Many running stores will let you take the shoes out for a run before you buy them; to make sure they're a good fit. You could also run around the store to get a feel for the shoes before you purchase them. Likewise, many will allow you to return a pair of shoes, even if you've worn them for several runs, if you find they're not working for you. The wrong running shoe can cause injuries, so most sports stores are happy to accommodate you.

Knowing whether or not you over- or underpronate will be helpful information when you go to buy your shoes, as this information will eliminate a whole slew of potentials. Knowing how many miles you plan to run per week is also good information. There's no need to buy the top-of-the-line running shoe and shell out over a hundred bucks if you don't plan on running more than five to ten miles per week. A less expensive pair will suit you just as well, and save you some money in the process. Beyond that, it's very much a matter of preference. Bring along a pair of thin running socks and try on a whole bunch of shoes—they all feel quite different. Some will make you feel like you're floating on air, and others will feel awkward. But when you find the right pair, you'll generally know it. You'll slip on the shoes, they'll hug your foot perfectly, and you'll know you found the pair for

QUESTION: **How often do you need to replace your running shoes?**
ANSWER: **Approximately every 300–500 miles of running.**

you. Here are some of the top names in running shoes. Buying a pair from any of these brands will serve you well: Adidas, Asics, Brooks, New Balance, Nike, Reebok, Rykä, Saucony.

Bring a friend with you for support when you go to make your purchase, and take your time making your choice. If you go to a nonspecialty store, and the employees don't know specifics for running shoes, hold off on making the purchase. My friend Amy went to buy a pair of shoes at a major sporting goods chain, and unwittingly relied on the salesperson's expertise, buying the expensive shoes the store recommended. After working out in the shoes a few times, Amy's feet were hurting, so she took the shoes back to the store only to find out that the shoes were intended for a completely different sport!

Running Clothes for Women

As I mentioned in the chapter outlining benefits of running, one of the great things about this sport is that you don't need any fancy clothes to run. A pair of solid running shoes and some comfortable clothes should suffice. But if you're going to make a commitment to running, there are a couple of staple clothing items that you'll want to introduce to your closet.

I'll take this opportunity to voice one of my major frustrations among the sporting goods industry. There just aren't a whole lot of options out there for women at the major sporting goods chains. Many of these stores have entire departments devoted to various men's sports—basketball, hockey, boxing, football, soccer. And then when you ask for the women's section they lead you to a little carousel in the corner of the store with a haphazard collection of running bras and shorts. When I'm in these stores I always make it a point to inquire as to the unequal real estate and selection. One man working at a store actually told me that women would buy men's clothes, whereas men wouldn't buy women's clothes. And this was this man's explanation for why there wasn't more selection for women. How lame is that? Never fear—there are a couple of venues that cater to women and women's sports apparel, and I list these at the end of the chapter.

Running Bras

Running bras are extremely important to me, and I look for a bra that gives me good support and really pushes my chest close to my body so it doesn't move much when I'm running.
Bridget, 32

Running bras are something all women need to contend with. Most women have probably already worn these for other sports. A running bra will serve you well to keep your runs more comfortable for your breasts. Most bras are made of a combination of cotton and Lycra—that stretchy comfortable material that helps things fit snugly to your body. The best running bras are lined with CoolMax, Dri-Fit or Drylete to keep the part against your body as dry as possible. As you look for the right running bra, keep in mind that as aerobics and yoga continue to gain popularity, there are many "exercise" bras on the market that might not offer the true support of a running bra. Many name brands have exercise bras that provide more fashion than function. Check the inside of potential running bras for thick layers of supportive material, and try them to ensure a good fit.

Running bras come in all shapes and sizes, colors and patterns. Many women wear their running bras sans T-shirt in the hot weather, so they come in sporty prints and styles. Running bras can be a little pricey—ranging anywhere from $20 to $50 a pop, so you'll want to try on the bra before you buy it. Something I have a problem with is finding running bras that aren't too tight around my chest below my breasts where the thick elastic holds it all in. A too-tight fit is very constricting around my chest. Ideally, you'll want a bra that fits you snugly, but doesn't feel too tight in any one area. Here's a good test—if you need the help of a friend or partner to pull it off you, chances are it's probably not the right fit for you.

If you're a woman with large breasts (above a C cup), there are a number of running bras designed specifically for you. It's important that you find the right bra so you can avoid neck, back and shoulder aches while running. Here is just a sampling of what's available to enable you a comfortable run:

- Champion Action-Shape Sports Bras (above C cups)
- Athena Sports Top (sizes C–DD)
- Elite Empower Bra (sizes C–D)
- Bounceless Bra (sizes D, DD, E)

Shorts

Running shorts for women are few and far between. Remember my story regarding women wearing men's clothes? Well, two of my regular pairs of running shorts are indeed from the men's department, because the selection in the women's corner didn't suffice. When buying running shorts, you want to find a pair of loose, lightweight nylon shorts, ideally with a cotton brief built into the lining. The lining prevents your underwear from hanging out of the shorts, so you don't flash the world when you're stretching and running. You also want to make sure that the waistband on the shorts isn't too snug—again, you want your running clothes to be as comfortable as possible. Running shorts come in a variety of lengths as well, and depending on how they fall on your inseam, you may experience chafing along your inner thighs. Lighter, softer material tends to reduce the risk of chafing, and applying some Vaseline to that area prior to a run can be good preventative medicine.

> Dri-Fit, CoolMax, Drylete and other similar wicking fabrics are designed to keep your skin dry while allowing your sweat to pass through. These fabrics are strongly advised over cottons, as cotton tends to soak up sweat and prevent your body from staying cool and dry.

No use starting off a run with any comfort strikes against you. Running shorts range in price from $10 to $30.

Tights

If you live in a climate where the temperature drops below fifty degrees—which includes most of us—you'll want to invest in a pair of running tights. While you could run through the winter months with sweatpants, and many women do, running tights will give you the most comfort and flexibility, and will keep you warm and dry. Tights are usually made of a nylon/Lycra combination so they fit snugly and comfortably. Most have a zipper at the ankle and a drawstring around the waist so you can control how tight you want them to fit. When buying running tights, look for a pair that is made with CoolMax or Dri-Fit, or any other such fabric—again, the goal is to allow the sweat to exit your tights, while keeping your legs dry and warm. A decent pair of running tights will run you about $40 to $50, but luckily you'll only need one or two pairs. Tights are machine washable and should hold up season after season.

Tops

Unless you're wearing your running bra as your one and only top during your runs, you'll want some sort of outer layer, depending on what the weather is like. I tend to throw on simple lightweight tank tops or T-shirts over my running bras—tops I'd wear as a part of my nonrunning life. I do have a couple of traditional "running tops," which are extremely lightweight tops—available in tanks, short sleeves or long sleeves—made with CoolMax or Dri-Fit. These tops provide a bit of protection from the elements while still keeping you comfortable, cool and dry. One thing I would steer away from when running is heavy cotton sweatshirts and T-shirts. These don't breathe at all, and they tend to soak up your sweat—causing them to get heavier and not allowing for your internal thermometer to accurately regulate your body temperature.

You also may want to invest in a windbreaker of some sort, as these are lightweight and protect you from the wind and rain while not being too heavy or causing you to overheat.

I'm most comfortable running in as little as possible. I don't like sleeves on my shirts, or anything that feels restrictive.
Laurie, 31

When I'm training for a triathlon I usually run without socks so I can prepare my feet for race days when I won't have the time to put them on.

Eileen, 26

Socks

When I was running track in my freshman year at Penn State, I would go visit my fellow teammates Pam and Laurie in their dorm across campus. I could always spot their room from the other end of the hall because there would be two sets of running shoes plopped on the floor outside their door. They were outside rather than inside the room because they stank so much. Pam and Laurie ran without socks. I soon started to as well, because, well, Pam and Laurie did it, and I thought that was cool. Soon, my shoes stank to high heaven and, I too, would keep them out in the hallway to fend off the odor. My husband is probably very thankful that I have reverted back to wearing socks when I run. I don't remember how long ago I made the switch—I think when I started running longer distances. Either that or when I couldn't stand the smell any longer myself.

Odor aside, socks protect your feet and give you a more comfortable run. Just as in tops and tights, look for socks made from a fabric like CoolMax. These will allow your feet to breathe and help fend off blisters at the same time. If you're running shorter distances, a more standard cotton running sock will probably be fine, but whenever I run any long distance, I always wear thin, CoolMax socks.

Accessories for Runners

There are all kinds of accessories for runners, depending on what your needs are. They're all things that can sometimes enhance your running experience.

Watches

I usually run with a watch. It's part of my whole anal retentive thing—I generally like to know exactly how long it took me to go a certain distance so I can compare it with previous runs along the same route, figure out my mile pace and keep track of my times. Every now and then I'll go out for a run and say, "Forget it. No watch today." That is a freeing moment. To run without a watch can take pressure off and keep you more focused on enjoying the run.

That being said, most runners choose to run with watches, and there are plenty of runner's watches to choose from, although the Timex Ironman watch is probably the one used most by runners. Regardless of the brand you buy, you'll want to make sure that your running watch has a "chron" (short for chronometer), which is a timer of sorts for runners. Chrons usually have multiple functions: start, stop and lap. If you just want to time your run from start to finish, then use only the start and stop features on the watch. If you want to keep track of your time at certain intervals within your run, like half-miles or miles, the lap function will help you to do this. To use the lap function, press start at the beginning of your run. As you pass each interval marker, press the lap button. This will keep your lap time stored in memory, while continuing to keep track of your cumulative time, as well as recording the new "lap" time from zero. When you finish your run, press the stop button. Now, you have a detailed record of your run—interval by interval. To see your lap times, just press the lap button and it will run through all of your lap times for the entire run. Check how many laps your watch will store. Mine stores eight laps, while my husband's watch stores one hundred.

Usually in my shorts I'll have some money and a key, but I've never been a huge fan of having extra stuff with me when I run.
Beth, 35

Fanny Packs

There are many different types of fanny packs made specifically for runners. Some of them are small and are the perfect size to hold some keys, a couple of bucks, lip balm, and a gel pack or two for long runs. Your fanny pack will hook onto the waistband of your shorts or tights, and if you wear it on the back side of your shorts, you'll barely even know it's there.

Then there are what I call the "mega" fanny packs. I just started to run with one of these in the past month, as I realized it will help me get through this upcoming marathon. These more substantial packs are true fanny packs in that they go all the way around your waist and hook shut with a plastic fastener. These mega fanny packs usually come with a plastic water bottle, which rests nicely in a pouch along the back. Some have zippered compartments on either side of the bottle where you can keep all kinds of goodies. I used to think these fanny packs looked pretty cumbersome, and I like to run with as little extra weight as possible. But running in Southern California is much different than back East. There are no water fountains in many of the places I run these days, so I need to bring my own water. And it's warm enough out here that I need access to water throughout my entire run. Initially, I ran carrying a water bottle, switching hands back and forth as my carrying arm wore out. Talk about feeling bogged down. Hence, the mega fanny pack. Now I can have water anytime I want, and keep my hands free at the same time.

Running Vests

Running vests are great add-ons to your running wardrobe, as they are perfect for those days when you're not sure if you should be wearing long sleeves or short sleeves, jacket or no jacket. On days like this, I go for the lesser of the clothing options, and throw on a fleece vest over the top. It usually does me right. Most running vests have zippered pockets for storing gloves, keys or money.

Baby Buggies

One of the wonderful things about running is that you can share it with your baby. Running strollers or baby buggies are extremely popular, and come in all shapes and sizes—there are even double buggies for twins or two young ones. These are designed to give your baby a smooth ride while not interfering with your run by being overly cumbersome.

Nose Strips

You may have seen people running with a beige-colored strip across the bridge of their noses. No, it's not a Band-Aid. It's a nose strip, designed to keep your nasal passages open wide for optimal oxygen intake. I've worn these twice when running marathons, and they do what they say. If you've got a deviated septum, you might find these make a big difference in allowing you to take in more air through your nose.

Key Holders

Many running shorts and tights come with little key pockets in the inside near the waistband, but some runners like using little key storage cases that can be laced into the top of the running shoe. These are great because you don't feel the weight of the key jiggling around in your shorts. You won't even know your key holder is there.

Dressing for the Weather

The way I look at it is, it's never bad weather, it's just inappropriate clothing.
Lauren, 35

What the weather is like on any given day will determine how you dress, and what extras, if any, you'll need. When dressing to run, the key is to dress as lightly and as comfortably as possible, and to make sure you're warm enough that you don't develop hypothermia, and cool enough that you don't overheat. One of the most valuable things I learned along the way with regards to dressing to run is the "Twenty Degree Rule."

The Twenty Degree Rule dictates that you should dress for a run as if the temperature were twenty degrees (Fahrenheit) warmer than it actually is.

For example, if the current temperature is 55° Fahrenheit, and you're going to run, you should dress as if it's 75°. If you dress for 55°, you'll undoubtedly be too warm once you begin exercising. However, if it's cold outside and you're afraid of leaving the house with too little clothing, *dress in layers*. Bring the gloves and stick them in your tights once you're warmed up. Dressing in layers that you can take off and wrap around your waist is an easy way to ensure that you're never too hot or cold.

Warm Weather

No matter where you live, there will be times of the year when the weather will be very warm, and running outside will be difficult. Your best bet when running in warm weather is to try to keep your body as cool as possible. Wear lightweight, and light-colored, clothing. A running bra and shorts is sometimes enough. If you want to wear a top over your running bra, a tank made in a lightweight, breathable material will help keep you cool. If the sun is out in full force, you'll want to protect yourself by wearing sunscreen, and some sort of sun visor or hat (one with a mesh or vented top is best).

Cold Weather

Thankfully for me, the days of cold weather running on a regular basis are over. But I did run outdoors year round in New York, and I have fond memories of trying to shelter my face from the biting cold wind in the middle of February, and spending an entire run trying to catch gargantuan snow flakes in my mouth. Running in the dead of winter can actually be great—having a park all to yourself with the snow falling softly on the trees can be a very peaceful thing. As long as you come prepared.

When I run in the winter, I have a pretty typical ensemble. It goes something like this: shoes, socks, running tights, nylon running pants on top of the tights (if it's *really* cold, as in a windchill factor in the twenties), a Dri-Fit long-sleeve running top with collar, a long sleeve shirt layer (more than one if it's *really* cold), thick cotton or fleece shirt, windbreaker jacket on the outside of it all, gloves, and a wool hat. Phew. As you can imagine, it takes me a while to get ready for a run in the cold, and even longer to get out of this getup when I'm done. If you're layering clothes for a winter run, layer in the following way, starting with what's closest to your body: 1) CoolMax or other such fabric long-sleeve top and bottoms (this will keep you dry even though you're sweating), 2) cotton layer (thick or otherwise), 3) nylon windbreaker (this should always be the outside layer as it will prevent the cold chill from reaching your skin).

When it's really cold outside I always make sure to cover up my head and my hands. If I can keep them warm, I'm usually okay.
Emily, 29

Running in the Rain

This is something you might be surprised to find you enjoy doing. I know I enjoy running in the rain, *on occasion*. There's something very peaceful about schlepping through puddles and being one of the few people on the sidewalk without an umbrella. And the warm shower and dry clothes after your run will never be more rewarding. Make no mistake—if you run in the rain you will get wet. But I've found if I can keep the rain off of my face, everything else is bearable. I always wear a baseball or running hat of some sort with a brim large enough to shield my face from raindrops. And if you're standing outdoors in the rain waiting for a run or race to begin, trash bags with a hole poked in the bottom can make great makeshift rain slickers.

Running Apparel—Focus on Women's Wear

Thankfully, there are several companies out there that cater to the women's sports and running market by creating clothes made *by women for women*. There are yet other retail outlets geared toward outfitting the women athlete. Here are a few of the best resources for women's running gear.

Moving Comfort

Moving Comfort is probably the biggest name in women's fitness clothing made by women for women. Moving Comfort was founded by Ellen Wessel and Valerie Nye in 1977 in part as a response to the realization that nobody was making clothes for women. Women found themselves running in clothes designed for skinny men. Over the years, Moving Comfort has become the top name in women's-only sports apparel. Their website explains what makes women's athletic wear different from men's: *"Compared with men, women are generally broader in the hips, and narrower in the waist. Our rises (the distance between the waist and crotch) are generally longer. Our arms are proportionately shorter. Our backs are narrower. A good fit is a prerequisite for comfort and freedom of movement."* Moving Comfort does not have a catalog, but you can find their products in major stores like REI and Nordstrom, among others. You can also order Moving Comfort clothes through Title 9 Sports catalogs (see below). Moving Comfort also has a website that lists retailers that sell their clothes near you: See *www.movingcomfort.com.*

Lioness

Lioness was founded in 1992 by runner Renita Wallack. Like Moving Comfort, Renita started the clothing line to fill a void in women's running clothes on the market. The Lioness website (*www.lionessrun.com*) offers a list of retailers where their clothing is available, as well as online ordering capability.

Title 9 Sports

Title 9 Sports is one of my favorite retailers of women's running clothes. The company's tag line is *Clothing Inspired by and Cre-*

ated for Women. All of the women in their catalog "modeling" the clothes are real women, real athletes. Not world-class athletes or professionals, but real women. You know—*Jane, a 40-year-old nurse from Seattle.* That kind of thing. Just flipping through the catalog is very inspiring to see the photos of real women enjoying the heck out of exercising. Title 9 Sports was founded in 1989, and is based in Berkeley, CA. They feature many different brands of clothing (including Moving Comfort), and you can find everything from running bras to shoes to swimsuits to underwear to running shoes. Check them out at *www.title9sports.com*, or call them at 800-342-4448 to request a catalog. Their website features a lot of great information, including how to figure out what size running bra will work best for you.

Rykä

Rykä is the first line of fitness shoes made just for women. While I haven't tried these out, they have a line of running shoes that has received rave reviews. Visit their website at *www.ryka.com*

Ultimately, when dressing to run, the key is comfort. I have a friend who runs in her pajamas some mornings, because it was the easiest and most comfortable choice for her on that day. Try a variety of running clothes on different runs. You'll eventually settle on those that most make you feel good about yourself, while keeping you comfortable throughout your entire run.

I motivate myself by making sure that I've got good shoes and clothes that I like to run in. Clothes that make me feel like I look good when I'm running.
Sarah, 28

4

Keep It Loose:

The Importance of Stretching

I am always amazed when I meet a runner who says she doesn't stretch, either before or after a run. More often than not, it is men, not women, who tend to skip this essential aspect of any fitness routine. But it is surprising how many people consider stretching to be an ancillary "exercise." It's not. In fact, stretching is considered by many health experts to be as crucial to overall fitness as aerobic and anaerobic exercise.

For me, I turned stretching into a genuine component of my workout. Back in New York, it was one of many favorite parts of my run. You see, I used to have a *stretching tree* in Central Park. Some people use floor mats. Some use rope. Others stretch with a partner. But for many years, I couldn't begin any run without first leaning up against this huge old oak tree at the 90th Street entrance to the park. I would impatiently hang out by the neighboring kiosk if someone else was using the tree for a similar purpose. When it was finally free, I would step up,

I stretch after a workout and sometimes during, because flexibility is a critical part of fitness, and I know it's the reason why I have remained largely injury free.
Gail, 52

place my right foot on a nub of root jutting out of the ground, and lean in with all my weight to stretch my calf. Switch feet. Next came the hamstrings. Then my thighs. Muscle by muscle, I used the tree to complete my routine and get ready for my run. By incorporating this tree into my "ritual," I ensured that I always got in the necessary stretches before a run. At the same time, I had a familiar and strong icon to mark the start and finish of each workout.

Since I've moved to California, one of my running partners from back home told me that my stretching tree is no longer accessible. Apparently the park commission is relandscaping the 90th Street entrance, and they chained off the tree and the dirt around it. This makes me sad. That tree was where Frank and I met before runs. That's the tree Derin and I stood under waiting for the rain to pass, eventually deciding to ditch the run and go home and order Chinese food. That's the tree that houses a family of raccoons, one of whom scared me to death one night as I leaned into the tree and looked up only to find myself face-to-face with the furry thing.

My cats sometimes crawl all over me when I stretch. Stretching just feels so good. It feels the way yoga feels.
Christie, 29

Here in California, I haven't found anything that quite matches up to that big old tree. Before morning runs, I do my stretching in the living room, dirtying up the wall in the hallway with my shoes and using the couch as a prop. At the Hollywood Reservoir, I do my pre- and post-run stretching with the help of the bridge that goes across the dam. While none of these newer rituals has the same personal calming effect of my tree back in New York, they are still a part of my running experience. I don't even think about the stretches anymore—my body just kind of moves from one stretch to another, as if it's memorized the routine.

The Importance of Stretching

Out of all of the things you can do good for your body—lift weights, run, eat well—flexibility is the key to good health and preventing injury as we get older. According to the American Council on Fitness, stretching is good for our bodies in many ways:

- Allows greater freedom of movement and improved posture
- Increases physical and mental relaxation
- Releases muscle tension and soreness
- Reduces risk of injury
- Improves circulation
- Helps with coordination
- Reduces anxiety and stress
- Synchronizes mind and body

I never run without stretching my calves because I tore one playing tennis, and now they're just a little bit weaker than the rest of my body.
Laura, 36

Stretching Techniques

Watch some people stretching and you'll notice they bounce up and down. This is not the person to model your stretching technique after. While years ago this was considered an acceptable way to stretch, common knowledge today dictates that the safest and gentlest way to stretch is to slowly move into the position, and hold it. Once you're in the position, inhale deeply. As you slowly exhale, move into the stretch a bit deeper if possible, and if desired. Then hold this new position for ten seconds or so. You might even want to move farther into the stretch one more time. Keep your breathing steady, deep and slow. But remember—*stretching should not hurt.* Sure, some stretches are a bit uncomfortable because they're challenging achy muscles to do things they may not have done in a long time. But there's a good pain and a bad pain. The good pain (a slight discomfort) is expected, and any runner at any level will feel this type of pain when they reach their own personal threshold. But sharp, serious pains should not be the norm. Sharp pains may also be a sign that you've moved beyond stretching the muscle itself to the ligaments protecting the muscle. Stretching ligaments can make you more susceptible to strains and sprains.

STRETCHING DO'S AND DON'TS

Do	Don't
Slowly move into the stretch and hold	Bounce as you stretch
Stretch to the point of mild discomfort	Stretch to the point of sharp pain
Inhale deeply and exhale fully, mid-stretch	Hold your breath
Stretch both sides of your body evenly	Focus on only one half of your body

When to Stretch

A question I get asked a lot is when is the best time to stretch—before or after a workout? My answer is always the same—both. It's always good to do some light stretching before working out, to help warm up the muscles. You're less likely to injure yourself by pulling or straining a muscle if you've done a good job of warming up first. On the same note, stretching after a workout is just as important. In fact, it is widely thought that postworkout stretching is more beneficial than preworkout

I stretch before and after, and then more after. And I like to walk a little bit after I run, too.
Sarah, 26

because it helps reduce the buildup of lactic acid in your muscles, and ultimately prevents soreness. Have you ever done aerobics or some similar activity, and when the instructor said, "Make it burn," you really felt that burning sensation? That burning is caused in part by lactic acid in the muscles. Stretching and cooling down keeps that lactic acid moving through and out of your body rather than nestling in your quadriceps for an overnight stay.

I stretch after my run. I feel so good after I run and it's a time to do deep breathing and get in touch with my body.
Michele, 33

Feel free to stretch *during* exercise, too. My husband and I both suffer from iliotibial band syndrome (ITBS), and it can cause a painful tightening in the outside of the hip or knee socket. So on days when we're doing longer runs, we stop

Lactic acid forms in the muscles during intense anaerobic activity, and when it builds up it leaves your muscles feeling achy and sore.

and stretch as needed to keep that band loose and fend off the pain. We look forward to these breaks during really long runs, and they often do more than just keep us loose—they give us the *oomph* we need to get through the rest of our run. *Listen to your body.* If you're running and you feel a cramp in your hamstring or in your calf, don't ignore it. Stop and stretch it out. It won't take away from any of the benefits of your run, and it will prevent injury.

Stretching is one of those things you can never do too much of (like sit-ups), and you can gain benefits from stretching even on your nonrunning days. And if you have a problem area, stretching on days that you don't run can be just as, if not more, beneficial than stretching on your running days.

I have a tendency to really focus on my prerun stretching and then, depending on my time constraints, skimping on my postrun stretches. If it's cold out and I've just done a long run or a race—something where I really pushed myself and I'm exhausted—I've even been known to come home and plop down on the couch under a blanket and take a two-hour nap. If I did this without stretching between the end of my run and my collapse on the couch, I can pretty much guarantee that I'm going to be stiff and sore as hell when I wake up. While a little stiffness after a hard workout can actually seem like a good pain (it reminds you that you did something positive for yourself), if it affects the way you walk down stairs or forces a groan out of your mouth every time you lower yourself into a chair, then it's not such a good thing.

So. No matter how little time you have or how much you dislike stretching, make sure you build it into your running routine. A typical pre- or postrun stretching routine should take only five to ten minutes. And if you're short on time and have to cut into your stretching time, your after-run stretch is more important. If you don't stretch prior to a run, just take it easy when you start and use a slow jog at the beginning as your actual warm-up.

Stretching is a lot like yoga in many ways—it's a way for us to get in tune with our bodies and spend some quiet, quality time with ourselves and our physical beings. It's a very nurturing experience. If you have the time after a run, sit down on the ground, whether on the grass in the shade of a tree or on your carpet in the living room, and spend some time thanking your body. Close your eyes and breathe deeply into your

I do my stretching at night before I go to bed. That way I don't get muscle aches in the middle of the night.
Paulette, 50

For me, stretching is kind of that quiet time that says I'm preparing myself for what I'm about to do. I find it's a time to focus my mind and get my body ready to go.
Karen, 39

If you are short on time and have to cut into your stretching routine, skip the prerun stretch and focus on the postrun stretch.

After a run, I usually do a full body stretch and make a mental note of how I feel at that moment.
Shareena, 32

stretches, holding them for a moment longer when you're ready to release from a stretch.

Running Stretches And Techniques

Calves/Shins

Many women I know have problems with this part of the leg, often because the calves are underdeveloped. Calves are a very difficult muscle to build, and most women with muscular calves have their parents to thank. I am one of those big-calved women (although I can't find boots big enough to zip over my calves, so I don't know how thankful I am!). Because many women tend to run on their toes—this is especially true for runners who used to be sprinters or ran in short, quick spurts for other sports—this muscle can get strained easily. Tight calf muscles after a run can be terribly painful, especially when negotiating stairs. These stretches, when done both before and after a run, should prevent tight calf muscles. They'll also help to prevent shinsplints and Charley horses (described in chapter Nine).

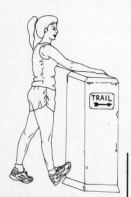

Lean and Lunge, Version 1
Keep your right leg straight, and place the front half of your foot against something perpendicular to the ground (a wall, a tree, a telephone pole). Lean forward as you concentrate on keeping your right foot flexed. Change sides.

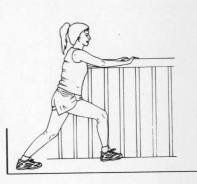

Lean and Lunge, Version 2

Bend your right leg at the knee, keeping the shin perpendicular to the ground, and your right foot flat. Stretch your left leg back and lunge forward, steadying yourself with a fence or tree. Change sides.

Hip Flexor

Women need to pay particular attention to stretching the hip area, because the way many of us run leaves the hips more susceptible to injury. These hip flexor stretches are a great way to hone in on the area around the hip socket, as well as the iliotibular band, a fibrous band connecting the outside of the hip socket with the outside of the knee joint. Here are some good hip stretches:

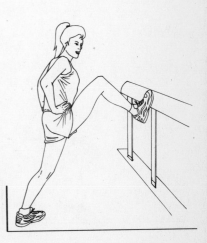

Bent Leg

Bend your right leg at the knee, and place your foot on an object about waist high (or higher). Keeping your left leg straight, lean into the elevated leg. Change sides.

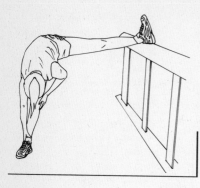

Side L

Place your left foot on an object about waist high, keeping leg straight and parallel to the ground. Bend forward at the waist, leaning down toward your right foot. Change sides.

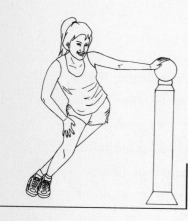

Crossed Leg

Cross your left leg in front your right leg, with your feet next to each other. Using a wall or tree to steady yourself, lean deeply into the left hip. Change sides.

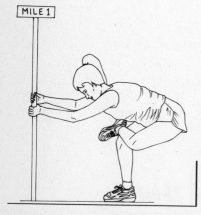

Sitting Cross-Legged

Bend your right leg, and place your left ankle on your right knee, as if you were sitting down in a chair cross-legged. Using a wall or fence to keep your balance, sit deeper into the stretch, making your bent left leg parallel to the ground. Change sides.

Quadriceps

The quadriceps, that bulk of muscles at the front of the thigh, is the largest group of muscles in the leg. These muscles, along with the knee joint they connect to, can take a pounding when running, especially when going up or down steep hills. Properly stretching this muscle can help prevent cramping or tightness in the thighs during and after runs.

I know that I'm supposed to stretch because of the benefits, but for me, it's more for enjoyment than anything else.
AnneMarie, 32

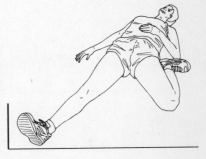

Bent Knee Hurdle
Sitting on the ground, bend your right leg back placing your foot next to your butt, and keep your left leg extended straight. Gently lie back and relax. Change sides.

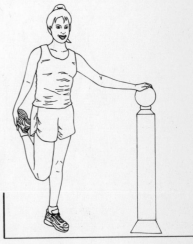

Foot in Hand
While standing, steady yourself, bend your left leg behind you as if to kick your butt, and grab your foot with your left hand. Gently pull your foot toward your back. Change sides.

Hamstrings

Hamstrings are the muscles that run along the back of the leg from the top of the knee to the back of the butt. This muscle can get very tight very easily, and can cramp up if running up a lot of hills or for exceedingly long distances. We don't use this muscle very intensely in our everyday lives, so when pushed to the max, it can react strongly.

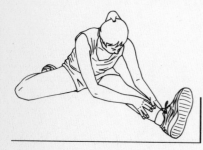

The Hurdle
Sitting on the ground, bend your left leg at the knee placing your foot next to your butt, and keep your right leg fully extended. Slowly lean forward. Change sides.

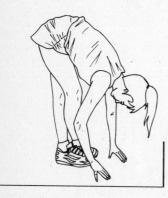

Bent Waist
While standing, cross your left leg over your right leg, with your feet right next to each other. Slowly lean forward toward the ground. Change sides.

Ankle/Foot

Runners often overlook stretching the ankle joint. Perhaps I'm especially conscious of this area because of my ankle break several years ago. Once I started running again, I had a great fear of twisting my ankle on rocks or other obstacles on the path, even though I had done exercise after exercise to strengthen my ankle and foot. However, I still always loosen my ankles before taking off for a run. The more flexible I am, the better the chances that my ankle and foot will roll with the bumps, so to speak.

If I'm short on time, I need to get out there and go. And then I work in the stretching afterwards while I'm doing other things. Like I'll step on the curb and stretch my calf.
Sarah, 28

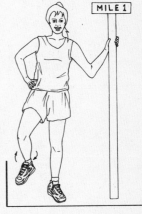

Ankle Rotation
Steadying yourself with a tree or wall, lift one foot off the ground, and slowly rotate the ankle in a circular motion, changing direction after several rotations. Change sides.

Arms/Shoulders/Back

Why would anyone need to stretch their arms and shoulders before a run? Aren't the legs doing all the work? Actually, the shoulder area is prone to muscle cramps because of the way we swing our arms and hold our backs and shoulders while running. I can get shoulder cramps pretty intensely at times, and they can

I wish I could spend more time stretching in the mornings, but I'm always rushed. On the weekends, I will absolutely spend 10 to 15 minutes stretching and really enjoy it.
Christie, 29

be as debilitating as any leg cramp or side stitch. One way to prevent these cramps is to do a few simple upper body stretches. I often do these as I'm doing my calf and shin stretches (a great way to save a few minutes if you're running late).

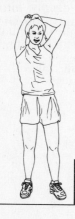

Shoulder

Bend your right arm and put behind your head as if to scratch your back. Grab your forearm or elbow with your left hand, and gently pull toward the left. Change sides.

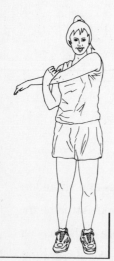

Triceps

Keep your left arm straight and cross it in front of your chest. Loosely grab hold with your right hand, and gently pull the straight arm toward your body. Change sides.

I know women who say that stretching is their favorite part of running and exercising. They're able to enjoy the way it feels, and splendor in the quiet time it provides them. Give yourself a chance to see if you're someone who can appreciate this time. Spend an extra long time stretching before, and more important, after, your run one day when you're not rushed for time. Focus on every little muscle, and breath deeply into the stretches. You may find this time is a calming and spiritual one for you, too.

Normally I spend about 20 minutes before I go to bed stretching my legs and my core. It feels great and I love knowing that I'm getting rid of toxins in my body.
Eileen, 26

5

Take It in Stride:

Beginning Your Running Program

My sister, Michele, was a walker. Thanks in part to Oprah's *Make the Connection*, every morning she got up at 5:30 A.M. and headed outside for a long walk with her dog, Willie. A couple of years ago, she decided to try running for a few minutes in the middle of her walk, with the hope that she would eventually build up to running her entire workout. She called me that afternoon from work with a lot of questions, the biggest one being "Why do you love to run so much?" "My heart was pounding so hard, I had to stop," she said. "And my shins hurt," she added. "It just felt so terrible. Is it supposed to feel that way?"

Well, yes and no. In this chapter we'll go through running, from the very first steps, to give you an idea of what it should feel like, both physically and mentally, so you can get started on your own running program with confidence.

Running was something that was hard when I first started, but I could do it at my own pace. It wasn't about running faster or longer . . . it was just about running.
AnneMarie, 32

The Basic Mechanics of Running

If you've never run before, you might not know where to begin, especially when it comes to exactly what our bodies should be doing. We all need a starting point. So I say, begin with what feels most natural for you, and we'll go from there. We've all run at some point during our lives, whether it's running down the street to catch the bus or playing freeze tag with the kids down the street. Running has been described as the most natural form of cardiovascular exercise there is.

For me, running is my stress break, my time to get out. I teach, so it's a break from the kids just to get out and clear my head. Karen, 25

I've found that the key to running efficiently (and in a way that feels good to boot) is to make sure that all the different parts of your body are working together toward the common goal—running. Ideally, you want to make the most efficient use of all of your muscles and body movements, so that running is a fluid, stress-free exercise for you. There are a couple of different areas to focus on, so we'll break them down, body part by body part. They are:

- Arms
- Shoulders
- Waist
- Head
- Hands
- Knees
- Feet
- Breathing

Arms and Upper Body

When I was in high school, I ran winter track as a way to get in shape for spring track. Because the length of an indoor track is smaller than a traditional one, I raced the 600-meter dash, a race that had me doing three laps along a 200-meter track at top speed. I remember my coach (the same one who told me I was getting chunky) standing alongside one of the turns, yelling for me each time around to relax my shoulders. And each time I heard his voice, I would realize my shoulders had tensed up and I would consciously focus on dropping them loose.

I still often find myself tensing up my shoulders when I'm running, especially if I'm running fast or uphill. But ideally, everything in your upper body should be relatively relaxed while you run. Again, the goal is to expend as little energy as possible on anything physical that isn't directly related to running. For example, when I'm running, my face is deadpan, expressionless. I take care not to tense the muscles in my face by gritting my teeth or squinting my eyes. I realized this when I ran on a treadmill in a hotel that had a mirror plopped right in front of the machine. For thirty minutes I observed the skin on my face bouncing up and down—it looks pretty funny.

I see people run with their hands balled up in fists. I feel like if I can keep my hands loose, I can keep my body loose.
Christie, 29

Working your way down, your shoulders and arms should be relatively relaxed, too, all the way down to your fingertips. In other words, don't run like Carl Lewis with your hands tensed, all five fingers splayed out. It looks cool, but you won't get any benefit from this except for, well, looking kind of like Carl Lewis when you run. Try to keep your shoulders dropped low, with your arms swinging comfortably at your sides, bent slightly at the elbow, and hands loose and hanging. The only time you'll want to really use your arms is when you're running up a steep hill. Using your arms and concentrating on pumping them will force your legs to go along with them. But for the most part, your arms should play little role in your run, other than keeping you balanced and coordinated. There is actually a world-class woman marathoner who lets her arms hang limply at her side, so they actually flail about as she's running. I was intrigued after seeing her run, and tried her technique sometime later that week. For me, it felt really weird and unnatural (and it looked kind of strange, too). The most important thing is to go with what feels right for you, remembering that the key is to stay as relaxed as possible.

I assumed that when I first started running, I could just go out and run a couple of miles and that would be it. And I was so disappointed that after a mile I died. So I started running little distances every day.
Paulette, 50

> **UPPER BODY RUNNING FORM HIGHLIGHTS:**
> - **Keep face relaxed**
> - **Drop your shoulders**
> - **Have arms swinging comfortably at your sides**
> - **Slightly bend at the waist**

With regards to your upper torso as a unit, the top half of your body should be bent ever so slightly forward at the waist, almost as if you're leaning forward in the direction you want to be going. You shouldn't lean over so far that it looks like you're actually in the midst of tripping forward, because you want to keep your air passage opened and unrestricted, but just enough so that the leaning of your upper torso naturally propels you forward.

Running Stride and Lower Body

I ran in a big group run yesterday, and knowing I was in the process of writing this chapter, I distracted myself from the task at hand (running), by observing my corunners' forms. I came to the grand conclusion that no two runners run alike. Everyone's got his or her own thing going on. Some people looked like they were struggling with every step—pounding their feet, moving their arms wildly, kicking their heels way up in the air, bobbing their heads up and down like an apple in a tub of water. And yet others glided forward with such little movement that you'd barely know they were running except for the fact that they were going in a forward direction with some speed. This latter group of runners ran with their feet barely lifting off the ground and their progression looked truly effortless.

I try not to focus on stride size because I'm small. And I keep it at a pace where I can carry on a conversation with someone.
Emily, 29

Stride describes the distance between your feet with each running step, and how quickly you take these steps.

A lot of people refer to their "stride" when talking about running. This is just a way of describing your running steps. Again, our bodies already know how to run, so we all have a natural running stride. Going with the same notion of efficiency, something to avoid doing when running is grossly overstriding (running with your steps really far apart) or understriding (running with your steps too close together). Either of these techniques would make your body work harder to run.

My legs get tired first. I always think they're going to give out. But I keep going, because I have a pretty strong will.
Alice, 34

A good way to find out if your lower body is doing its job in running efficiently is to ask a friend to watch you run in your normal stride. Ideally, your head should remain relatively level as you run—so while your legs and feet are obviously moving quite a bit down there, your goal is to have your head stay at about the same level and not bob up and down too much. A bobbing head usually means that you're bouncing with your steps, and that's another form of wasted energy. Any energy used to go up and down is energy that you're not using to go forward, and going forward is what running is all about.

As you step forward, try to keep your feet relatively close to the ground. Your heels shouldn't kick up real high behind you, and your knees shouldn't come up too high in the front. Limit the movement of your legs to a point where your steps feel natural and relaxed.

Something women are particularly prone to is running with their feet landing directly one in front of the other. Picture a runway model—they almost cross their feet in front of each other with every step they take. Many women (myself included) naturally run with their feet falling in a straight line, probably because our center of gravity is lower than men's and we have these things called hips. I didn't know I was guilty of running like this until I ran along a painted white line in Central Park. I realized that my feet landed directly in the center of the five-inch wide line. So I started making an effort to have my feet land on either side of the white line, something that initially felt somewhat unnatural, but in a good way. I still have to remind myself of this tendency sometimes, but over the course of the past few years I have been able to make a change in my running stride for the better.

With swimming I have a natural stroke. With running, I've had to work much harder to develop that sense of flow.
Libby, 41

LOWER BODY RUNNING FORM:

- **Avoid kicking heels and knees up high**
- **Keep your feet close to the ground**
- **Stride shouldn't be too long or short**
- **Feet should be directly underneath hips**

Breathing

When I first started running, it was torture. It took me a long time to get the breathing correct. My limbs were okay, but learning how to catch my breath right was hard.
Laura, 36

How we control our breathing when running can make our experience easier or more difficult. I only became tuned in to this about seven years ago. I used to get side stitches (sharp, painful cramps in my side) when I ran, especially during runs where I was pushing myself, like speed workouts or races. If you've never had a side stitch, let me tell you—they can be pretty intense. When I started running with the UN Running Club, Coach Jorge told me to try breathing in through my nose and out through my mouth. He assured me this would regulate my breathing and heart rate even when it's elevated, and would help to prevent side stitches.

I tried this new technique on my next couple of runs and at first it felt pretty strange. Sometimes I didn't feel like I was taking in enough oxygen, so I'd go back to breathing in and out through my mouth. Other times I would space out a few minutes into my run and slip back into my usual way of breathing. But I kept working on it, and it's now my standard breathing pattern. Jorge was right—my instances of side stitches have become few and far between, and when I do get them, I'm usually able to run through them. Today, when I'm running a road race, I often revert back to breathing in and out of my mouth until I've found my comfortable race pace, and also when I'm trying to speed up at the end for my kick and I need to get more oxygen into my body. But generally speaking, breathing in through the nose and out through the mouth is

The best breathing form is to inhale through the nose, exhale out the mouth.

I never get out of breath during my everyday runs, and I think it's partly because I've been running since I was young, so my breathing pattern is really natural to me.
Bridget, 32

the simplest way to regulate and control your breathing when you're running.

How Running Will Feel

Running is a big unknown for many women, and there is always the fear of "doing it wrong," especially if this is your first time running. So, what will running feel like for you? There is no way I can correctly answer that question for you. Running is an extremely personal thing. For some, it may feel like you're trying to tap dance when all you've done your whole life is ballet. It may feel awkward, goofy, and just plain old strange. For other women, especially those who have run as part of another sport somewhere along the way, it may feel comfortable immediately. If you're in the former group, don't give up! Running is a lot easier than tap dancing, and after a few times out, you'll start to discover some moves of your own.

I remember those days when kids would make fun of me. "Can't you go any faster than that?" Paulette, 50

But before I go any further, I want to be blunt about something: *running sometimes feels like crap.* Invariably during any given run, I'll go through a stage, usually in the first mile or two, where my body makes no bones about its discomfort at the prospect of running. It's at this point that I'll have to convince myself to keep going with the belief that it will get better. In talking with other women runners, it seems that I'm not alone in this internal struggle. But I've found that it's the very process of getting through and moving beyond this point where the run feels so terrible that makes running so wonderful. Triumphing over feelings of doubt and discomfort to keep on going makes the end of a run all that much sweeter.

Usually it's not my legs that give out on me. It's my lungs.
Maggie, 25

Your breathing and heart rate are probably the first things that will affect you as you run. For the first few minutes, or even the first mile or two, your breathing will become irregular as it tries to adjust to the new task at hand and find a new rate to settle into. This is the point where most of us think to ourselves, "Hmmm . . . is it supposed to feel like I'm going to keel over?" But if you don't run too fast and you're not doing any major hills in your run, give your body a chance to adjust. And over time, your breathing should become more regular after a few minutes at its higher rate.

Your pace, or running speed, will have a lot to do with how good or bad your run feels. You'll have different paces for different runs. If you want to run a longer distance, perhaps a distance you haven't run before, you'll probably want to run at a slower pace to make sure you have enough energy to get you through to the end of your run. Whereas, if you're running a shorter distance or a race, you might want to increase your pace and push yourself a bit more.

When I started, I walked on the treadmill for a month and a half. Then I got the courage to go outside and I ran five houses. And every other day I added another house.
Sue, 55

My advice is to start by establishing what your own personal, comfortable jogging or running pace is. Run wherever you're most comfortable—on a treadmill, around the block, in a park. Begin your run at a pace that feels comfortable for you—not so slow that you feel as though you're holding yourself back, and not so fast that you feel fatigued and winded by the time you are finished and you couldn't go a step farther. Your goal is to discover your own pace and "groove"—a speed where your body is on board for your plan to run and doesn't give you too much resistance along the way. Another way to identify your comfortable pace is to run at a speed where you can converse with someone. If you're unable to talk at all while running, slow down. You're probably running too fast.

If it's convenient, you might want to consider taking a stopwatch to a track. Run two laps (a half-mile) or four laps (one mile) at your comfortable pace and use your stopwatch to time your run. If you run two laps, multiply your time by two, and this will be your mile pace, and if you run four laps, your finishing time will be your mile pace. To give you a general idea of how your pace fits into the bigger scheme, here is a general breakdown of mile paces for a 5K (3.1 miles):

- **5–6 minute miles = elite and fast runners**
- **7–8 minute miles = moderately fast**
- **9–10 minute miles = moderate**
- **11–12 minute miles = moderately slow**
- **12 + minute miles = slower runners**

Your pace is something that will change, depending on how frequently you are running, what distance you're running and what your goal is for the particular run. I'm training for a marathon right now, and my mile pace tends to fall somewhere around ten- to ten-and-a-half-minute miles. Yet, when I'm concentrating on a shorter distance like a 5K, I'll run between seven- and eight-minute miles. My morning runs with Derin and our friend Christie are usually run in a nine- or ten-minute mile pace. My point is, once you have an idea of what your comfortable base pace is, you'll have a point of reference so you'll know when you're pushing yourself more than usual, or when you could be comfortably pushing yourself a little harder. It may take you a month or two to become familiar with your base pace to a point where you'll know how different paces feel.

It's funny, 'cause I don't love it for the first ten minutes. But then everything kind of falls into place. Sarah, 26

When I'm running a lot, my body tends to "memorize" what different paces feel like and I can go out and run my miles within a few seconds of my target.

> 📖 **Mile pace** is the time it takes you to run a mile. This is a typical measuring method of speed and pace among the running community.

With every run, something in your body will usually start to signal your brain that it's time to turn around and go home, especially if you're running a longer than normal distance. For me, I've found there are three different things that could affect the length of my run, and how the run feels:

- Muscle and body fatigue
- Cramps or side stitches
- Cardiovascular fatigue

Muscle fatigue is that point you reach when your legs feel like bricks. When every step feels like you can't go on any farther. This type of muscle fatigue will usually affect me if I've run a longer than usual run over the weekend, and early the next week I go out for my usual five-mile run. On these mornings, even stepping off and onto curbs can be an effort.

Muscle and body fatigue gets us all at some point. Every now and then, your body will get tired of what you're putting it through and start sending your brain messages requesting that you stop. This is a natural part of running—if it wasn't, we'd just run and run forever. Sometimes I listen to my brain's request

The hardest thing for me was going from the treadmill to running outside. The treadmill keeps your pace and your time for you, and I still don't have timing down outdoors. Alice, 34

and stop. And make no mistake—stopping if you need to is absolutely okay. Other times I'm able to push through and run a little farther before calling it quits. Listen to your body and make the call that is the best for you.

Cramps and side stitches can sometimes cause you to stop a run short (they have shortened many of my runs over the years). I usually get cramps in two different areas: my sides or my shoulders. Cramps are a major inconvenience because they usually involve pretty sharp

RUNNING AND OUR BODIES

- If you've got long hair and are running on a hot day, expect your hair to become an entangled knot by the time you're finished. This is because of the bouncing motion of your hair against your sweaty neck and back. Try a braid or pigtails to avoid this.

- If you're premenstrual or menstruating, your breasts may be super sensitive at the start of a run. Make sure to wear an extra-supportive sports bra on these days, and a few minutes into your run the discomfort should go away.

- Some women experience a drop in body temperature after a run (myself included). This is because our internal cooling system has been working overtime to keep our body temperature regulated while working out, and sometimes it keeps working after we stop the run. Staying in wet, sweaty workout clothes can contribute to this chill. Get out of the wet clothes as soon as possible and take a warm shower.

pain that oftentimes won't go away until you massage the affected area, or discontinue the run. I talk more about side stitches in Chapter Nine; and give some suggestions as to how to get rid of them.

I just like to run at the crack of dawn at 6 A.M. when no one's on the street because it's really quiet and it gives me some time to think when I'm by myself. Pamela, 29

Lastly, there is **breathing and cardiovascular fatigue.** If you've been running hard and your breathing has been highly elevated, you may just reach a point where you need to stop running and catch your breath. Running in extreme conditions like humidity or cold weather can also affect your breathing and make each breath more of an effort while running. There are also certain times of the month that make breathing more difficult for us while running—particularly the week after ovulation (this generally coincides with PMS). Our heart rate is higher at this time, and so cardiovascular exercise feels more difficult.

When you reach any of these points of fatigue and what brings your run to an end depends on a lot of factors, including how far you're running, how rested your body is and so on. But the biggest variable here is you. The choice to run through the discomfort or cut it short is one you'll make many times. And there is no wrong choice to make.

Running for Beginners

Taking the First Steps

When I first started running, I agreed that I'd exercise for 45 minutes and would run two minutes at a time, with one minute of walking in between. Until I finally said, "Forget it. I'm going to see how far I can go."
Michele, 33

If you've never run before, there's no way to know what it's like unless you go out there and give it a try. Make sure you have a pair of running shoes (I explain how to select the right running shoe in chapter Three), some comfortable running clothes that are appropriate to the environment you're running in, and you're ready to go. For your first run, I recommend going somewhere flat and easy—a running track at a local high school or college, a park where there's some sort of paved or dirt path for runners, or even a treadmill.

Begin your workout with a warm-up. You wouldn't want to jump into an intense aerobics class without letting your body in on your intention and giving it a few minutes to adjust, right? The same applies to running. Ideally, you should spend several minutes warming up your muscles and heart rate, simply by walking briskly, and following with some stretching (see chapter Four). Warming up should be part of your usual routine, even after you've been running for a couple of weeks or months. You may find that it makes more sense for your warm-up to be slow jogging as opposed to brisk walking, if you're planning on an intense run. Keep in mind that the goal of warming up is to ease your body into the workout, so use your own common sense.

I run in the morning, so it starts my day off great.
Sue, 55

For example, if I were doing a slow run, a prerun stretch might be my entire warm-up. But if I were running in a race or were doing a speed workout, my warm-up would entail not only some prerunning stretches but some more traditional running warm-ups as well, such as slow jogging for a few minutes or some quick sprints—something to get my heart going and my muscles warmed up.

Once you're warmed-up, stretched and ready to go, start walking briskly. Then pick up your pace to a slow jog, and experience how running itself feels. As you continue to run, think about what's going on throughout your body. How do your legs feel? How about your feet? Is your breathing difficult? Do your arms feel natural swing-

WHEN NATURE CALLS

As a runner, all bets are off when it comes to things like spitting, blowing your nose and even peeing. The first time I blew my nose sans tissue in front of Derin, I was slightly concerned about the reaction I'd get. I mean, holding one nostril closed with your finger while blowing the contents of the other nostril out onto the ground is pretty gross. Derin didn't even blink. It's just one of those things that is acceptable, even expected, among runners. Peeing on the go is another. One mile into the New York Marathon in 1996, my friend Jeanette and I looked jealously at all the men peeing over the side of the Verrazano Bridge into the Hudson. What about our anxious bladders? A minute later, we ran over to the side of the bridge, dropped our shorts and squatted right there as the masses ran by. Looking around we saw we weren't the only ones. A strange memory, but there was no shame in having to do it. A girl's gotta do what a girl's gotta do.

ing at your sides? Try to keep your body as relaxed as possible as you experience this first run. You may want to set a goal for how long you want this first run to be—maybe it's two minutes. Maybe it's a couple of loops around a track. Maybe it's a mile. Whatever your goal, it's a good one, because it marks a starting point for making running a part of your life. Once you've achieved this first run, you'll have a base for every other run.

Setting Reasonable Goals

I love the fact that essentially anyone can be a runner. I don't think it takes some kind of innate skill.
Christie, 29

Setting reasonable goals is a really important part of any new running program, with the emphasis on "reasonable." I'm very much a believer in the attitude that our bodies and minds can achieve amazing things when working together, but it's important to set goals that are attainable and not too advanced at this early stage. Not achieving your first set of goals could be discouraging and act as a setback in your running. I suggest starting with something simple, like this:

Make running a part of my workout three days a week.

What do you hope to get out of your running program? Set a goal for your first eight weeks of running! My goal is to:

_____

_____

_____

_____

Whatever your goals are, keep them real to yourself and don't compare your progress to what your friends or other runners are doing. As I've said before, running is a very personal thing and all of our bodies have different reactions to it. Set your goals for yourself and don't worry if they don't sound too grand. You can continually set new goals as you build on your running foundation and running becomes a part of your life. Remember—the greatest rewards from running come from making it a regular activity. Be patient. You've got plenty of time to go longer and faster.

Scaling-Up Mileage

After you've been running consistently several times a week, the way to continue building up and growing is to lengthen the amount of time and distance that you run. This isn't something you should do quickly or in large chunks. Don't go from running ten minutes to running for a half-hour. However, I'm a firm believer in the idea that our bodies are capable of doing much more physically than we give them credit for, so gently pushing beyond our normal run times and distances can be a great thing. According to the Road Runners Club of America, new runners can expect to be able to jog for twenty continuous minutes within a month or two of beginning their running program.

In my experience, four weeks at any given distance is a reasonable amount of time to get comfortable and be ready for new challenges. So if your regular running distance is two miles, do that for about four weeks (three to four times a

I started running because I was having children and I wanted to be able to get outside and get some exercise that didn't involve driving to a health club. It needed to be easy.
Gail, 52

week), and then the next week, add on a quarter- or half-mile to one of your weekly runs. If you're running for ten minutes comfortably for four weeks, then add on two to five minutes to a handful of your runs. The goal is to keep expanding to a point where your intense cardiovascular workout is at least twenty to thirty minutes, so your body can take full advantage of what cardiovascular exercise has to offer. Be aware that increasing your distance too quickly at an early stage of running can make you more prone to injury, so take it slow. You've got the rest of your life to add miles!

Sample Weekly Workout Schedules

Here are a couple of sample workouts for different levels of beginning runners:

- **Group 1** = Those with no experience running

- **Group 2** = Those with some previous running experience

- **Group 3** = Occasional runners, or those who run as part of another activity

It's important to have down time. If you're not in the mood to run, you don't have to. I've realized over time that rest periods can be as revitalizing as running itself.
Beth, 35

Of course what follows are just guidelines, and you should use them to help you figure out what makes the most sense for where you are in your life and in your health cycle. Also, if you're currently not doing any sort of exercise, including walking, I suggest starting with a walking program, eventually building up the intensity and duration of your walks to a point where you're getting a cardiovascular workout from this activity. You can start adding in some jogging to your walks at that time.

The following workouts are based on running three or four days a week. If you're running three days a week, give your body a rest and don't do workouts two days in a row until you've built up a running foundation.

First 2–4 Weeks

3 x Week

GROUP 1:

Walk 3–5 minutes warm-up, run for 5–10 minutes, walk 3–5 minutes cool-down

3 x Week

GROUP 2:

Walk 3–5 minutes warm-up, run for 10–20 minutes, walk 3–5 minutes cool-down

3 x Week

GROUP 3:

Walk 1–3 minutes warm-up, run for 20–30 minutes, walk 1–3 minutes cool-down

Second 2–4 Weeks

GROUP 1:

4 x Week
> *Walk 3–5 minutes warm-up, run for 10–20 minutes, walk 3–5 minutes cool-down*

GROUP 2:

4 x Week
> *Walk 1–3 minutes warm-up, run for 15–25 minutes, walk 1–3 minutes cool-down*

GROUP 3:

4 x Week
> *Walk 1–3 minutes warm-up, run for 30–40 minutes, walk 1–3 minutes cool-down*

After two months of running, you can start to mix and match your workouts. Run longer distances on some days, shorter on others. Run some of your days faster and others nice and easy. *The idea in the first month or two is to make running a part of your life.* Acquire a taste for it, so to speak. Taking these first few months slowly is important in building a base, getting your body used to how running feels and ensuring your runs remain injury free. Ramp up only when you and your body are ready.

With two young kids, running was my chance to kind of get away, put my music on and find my time.
Karen, 39

Again, these workouts are suggestions only. The most important thing is to listen to your body. If you're supposed to run thirty minutes one day and you can't make it past fifteen, don't sweat it (no pun intended). You'll have other days when those thirty minutes feels great and easy, and you'll be tempted to run even more. Trust me. It will happen.

6.

All Dressed Up, Now Where to Run?

Finding Great Running Spots

For runners, the world is a virtual gym. Unlike many sports, you can really run anywhere. You don't believe me? Here's a story that I think of when I'm out of town and have convinced myself there's no place to run where I am. When I first graduated from college, I was working for the relief organization CARE, and went to Somalia during the peacekeeping mission there in 1993 to shoot a documentary. I spent my first week in the capitol of Mogadishu, staying in a small room at the CARE compound. Conditions in Mogadishu were very dangerous at that time, and the only thing between the twenty or so CARE staff members and the chaos of the city were the 20-foot-high cement walls of the compound and a handful of armed guards.

Now, if there were ever a valid excuse to cut back on a running routine, I would think this was it. But my first morning there, I woke up at five o'clock in the morning (jet-lagged and wired), and went outside to write in my journal and wake up. I

When I'm traveling, the first thing I do when I get there is map out my running route. I've run in some absolutely beautiful places— Paris, London, Hawaii.
Janet, 51

couldn't believe it when I saw one of the CARE staff members running laps inside the compound, one lap being about half the distance of a standard 400-meter track. Apparently he did this every morning, early enough to beat the heat of the rising desert sun. I'm sure he had many reasons for running inside the compound every day—keeping sane while his environment was so unpredictable probably being at the top of his list. But the image of this man running around that compound is something I've never let go of, and it reminds me that there's always a place to run, no matter where you are.

Granted, most of us will never be in a position where laps in an armed compound in a war-torn country is our only running option. Most of us have many choices when choosing where to run on any given day. And with a little creativity, and some street smarts, we can find running spots wherever we are. Here are just a few ideas:

- City parks
- Nature trails and off-trail running
- Road running
- Tracks
- Sidewalks
- Treadmills

I love running on the mountains, on the trails, and away from the city.
Karen, 25

Where to Run

City Parks

Parks can be paradises for runners, and a lifesaver for runners in urban areas. Most cities have a number of public parks that are large enough for a decent workout. Parks are ideal running venues, since many are already set up for runners and other sports enthusiasts, and offer maps highlighting running routes, mile markers, safety stations, and so on. Back in New York, my former Road Runners Club sells a map of Central Park that was invaluable. With the help of that map, I was able to put together all kinds of routes at varying distances, so I could pick and choose my running course each day, given any time constraints or muscle soreness I had. Check with the chapter of the Road Runners Club near you for information on parks in your community.

Another great thing about public parks is that they're usually set up for heavy public recreational use. Many are patrolled by local police or park rangers, making them a relatively safe alternative to running on the street or in remote areas. And you'll always find other runners sharing the park with you. And in-line skaters. And bikers. And walkers. And even the occasional cross-country skier on wheels. Running with all of these different people, whether just out to enjoy a beautiful day or seriously working out, is fun. It can be distracting, too (in a good way for me) to have such a variety of people to look at while you're running. Sometimes I spend an entire run reading the backs of people's T-shirts as they blow past me on their Rollerblades.

My favorite run is in Central Park. In the mornings I'd recognize people, and we wouldn't talk but we would nod and smile and acknowledge that we saw each other every morning. And that just made Manhattan feel like my home. Christie, 29

Parks have a natural infrastructure that's ideal for runners. If a park is well-designed, it will have water fountains scattered throughout—an important asset, especially during hot summer runs. Keep in mind that sometimes park departments turn these off during the winter months. Public bathrooms are another major benefit to park running. Many a time I've been running my standard loop in Central Park, and had to dash into the public rest room near the Boathouse there. This isn't a small consideration. It's no fun to be halfway through a run when an overwhelming urge takes over with no rest room in sight.

- **Does your park have a road running through it? See how many varieties of running courses you can create in your park.**

- **Need something to do when you're running? Count how many bridges and water fountains you see during your run.**

- **Put a spin on your run . . . run fast on the uphills, and slow on the downhills (or vice versa).**

- **Run your course in the reverse direction.**

The hardest part of my first race was this big hill in the park that I flew up, not knowing how much it would hurt my calves the next day. I just had so much adrenaline at the time.
Alice, 34

Lastly, parks can provide endless possibilities for workouts because of their very design. When my mom came to visit me after I first moved to New York, we went for a long walk through Central Park, which had since become my favorite refuge. I remember my mom exclaiming, "There's so much topography here!" I guess she had always envisioned Central Park as this big patch of green in the middle of Manhattan, and didn't realize it was intricate in design with hills, rocks and woods. Well, it's that same intricate design that makes Central Park and other parks rich training ground for runners. Central Park has several painfully steep hills—fine if you're running downhill, but daunting when you're at the bottom looking up. But, at the same time, they are perfect when I'm in the mood for a "hill workout" (described in chapter Eleven). Likewise, a nice curvy downhill can be a welcome relief a few miles (or a few hundred meters) into a run.

Nature Trails and Off-Trail Running

Nature and the great outdoors can present wonderful opportunities for new, fresh and revitalizing runs. This is no great secret. *Runner's World* magazine devotes a column each month to nature called "Rave Runs," where a hidden running treasure is photographed and presented, accompanied by a short quote from the runner who found the location special enough to write in to the magazine. The pictures have an almost spiritual feel to them, and make me want to dive right into the page and be in that place right then and there.

I didn't have any personal experience with true nature runs until a couple of years ago, when Derin and I drove up to Stowe, Vermont, for a long weekend in July. Our ultimate goal in this getaway was to escape the franticness of New York at a little bed-and-breakfast in beautiful surroundings. We chose Stowe largely because we read in a guidebook that there was a five-mile running trail weaving along a stream in the woods on the edge of town. We were able to pick up the trail about a hundred meters behind the B and B we were staying in.

I really enjoy running in the flats up by the Sierra Madres. There are a lot of stream crossings, and you've got shade and trees. I love it.
Lauren, 35

It was just what we needed. Running became one of the focal points of our weekend—we even planned some of our days around our runs because we wanted to take full advantage of this trail, which took us by brooks, over bridges, past fields of cows, encountering only the occasional biker or runner. Combine this scenery with crisp, fresh country air, and we were in runner's heaven. It was great to spend this quiet time with each other, bonding through the sweat, scenery and fresh air that surrounded us.

The running trail in Stowe was set up specifically for runners, so it was the ideal way to incorporate a little more adventure into our runs. But something that's becoming more and more popular these days is running "off-trail." This new trend in running is similar to mountain biking and other extreme sports. (When I say new, I really mean that the sport is becoming more mainstream, since even the first marathon in Greece was actually a form of off-trail running!)

Today, most shoe stores offer a variety of running shoes designed specifically for running off-trail. These shoes have a hip and rugged design to them, and some can even double for simple hiking shoes. If you're up for an outing of off-trail running, the world virtually becomes your path. Think about it . . . once you start looking at the great outdoors as opportunities for new running adventures, there is really no limit to where you can go, how tough or easy your workouts can be, and how many ways you can challenge yourself. And I have to say, running in less traditional running settings can be an incredibly liberating experience. I used to run along a horse trail that is uneven, muddy and full of twists, with occasional low-hanging tree limbs that I had to duck under. And sometimes I would hum the theme song to *Rocky* in my head as I turned and dodged. I felt cool. I felt like a jock. And feeling like a jock feels pretty good.

Bear in mind, off-trail running can present its own obstacles, the obvious ones being tree stumps, roots, rocks and the occa-

I think my favorite run is in the desert in Arizona. I had never been there before and I just went outside and ran. The best runs for me are when I don't know where the route is, and I'm just running it.
Maggie, 25

sional cobweb you'll plunge through. There are also the not-so-obvious concerns about off-trail running, specifically the wear and tear on the knees and ankles. Even small stones cause the runner's legs to react and over-compensate in an effort to protect the body, putting extra stress on the joints. There's also the issue of safety—trails can be isolated and present all kinds of special concerns for women, and therefore should never be run alone.

- Pick a new trail and run out for 10 minutes (or longer), and then turn around and run back. See how many things you notice on your way back that you missed the first time around.

- Run along a trail and pretend you're deep in the heart of the Costa Rican rain forest. Get "lost" in the surroundings.

- Drive to a state park, and try running on a hiking trail.

Does this mean you should stay away from off-trail running? Absolutely not. Just run smart. Even after my ankle break in 1996, I still venture off the beaten path. Just do what I do. Don't run too fast, and keep a close eye on what's coming up, being especially aware of roots and rocks in your path. And lastly, if you're going to run off-trail, find a running partner to go with you.

*I love running where I'm completely surrounded by nature, and where I can go for a really long time and I don't really have to think about how far I'm going, because I know that if I get to the end and turn around it's going to be a great run.
Bridget, 32*

Road Running

While the term *road running* can encompass running on many different surfaces, this section literally refers to running on the road. The street. Tarmac. Running on the road is a great option for runners who live in rural areas, where parks and tracks might be less accessible. It's also perfect for the runner who likes to chart her own course.

I did a lot of road running when I was in high school, since my cross-country team did all of its training on roads. My daily workout during those cool, fall days consisted of long runs on seemingly endless, one-lane country roads. We'd see only the occasional car during our forty- or fifty-minute run. Depending on who my running partner was that day (and how seriously they were approaching the workout), I'd stop to talk to the cows and horses at farms along the way. I've always been an avid animal lover, and found this little private time with the cattle quite calming.

Despite my occasional pit stops to get in touch with nature, my cross-country coach, Whitney Seltzer, must have known what she was doing by sending us out into the farmlands of Oley, Pennsylvania. She knew that once we committed ourselves to the run, we'd have to finish it in order to get back to the high school. This is a method I still use today. It's really foolproof—you only have to commit to the first half of any given run. Getting home takes care of the rest.

Since the road you're running on will most likely be free of any mile markers or other distance indicators, use natural icons along your way to help you measure your distance and speed, or just to give you some minigoals. I used to use telephone poles, fence posts, silos, streetlights, whatever, to keep my feet going. During those high school runs, I would invent little games for myself. I would run fast from one telephone pole to the next, and then I would slow down between that and the next one, and so on. This gave me something to keep my mind occupied, kept me moving forward, and made the runs fun. I didn't realize at the time that I was doing a form of interval training, which will be described in more detail in chapter Eleven. Road running can also offer some of the same benefits as running in a park, like encountering the occasional hill. Hills are beneficial in gaining running strength, which is a prerequisite to getting faster.

When road running, it's important that you pay particular attention to safety concerns (see chapter Nine). Run on the left side of the road, facing the oncoming traffic. And always make sure that there is an ample shoulder on the side of the road. Unless you're running along a one-lane country road like the one described earlier, it's important to stick to these rules.

Also, keep an eye out for loose pets. Now, I know that I've already expressed my love for animals and my habit of talking to them alongside of the road. But while visiting my parents-in-law in the foothills of the Sierra Nevadas, Derin and I had a scary encounter with a dog that reminded me of the considerations of rural running. After being spoiled to death by Derin's parents and spending a few days focusing on how much food we could ingest, we decided to redeem ourselves and go for a run along the small, windy roads leading to their house. About two miles into the run (and now of course, two long miles away from the house), we ran into a big, testy dog, vigilantly guarding its owner's farm. Now, I am a dog person. I mean, I LOVE dogs. But this dog, barking ferociously at us as we ran by, scared me half to death. And the dog was unleashed, with no fence or

- If you live in a rural area, walk out the front door, pick a direction and start running. See how many things you discover that you've never noticed before.

- Pick markers like telephone poles. Run from one telephone pole to the next. Then stop and walk to the next one. Then run to the next one. And so on.

- Run to work! Bring a change of clothes the day before and try running to work the next morning (provided you have a shower at work!).

anything else between this frothing animal and us. Luckily, Derin stared-down the dog while I ran along and the dog soon lost interest in us. My suggestion—if your run leads you to unfamiliar country roads without a lot of traffic, make sure to drive along your route first, and look for any potential trouble areas.

Local Schools and Tracks

If you're having trouble finding a good running place, try a track. Running tracks, whether at local high schools, colleges or parks, are an invaluable resource for runners. Most schools today have tracks, either made of a rubbery substance, a tarmaclike material called tartan, or cinder. But regardless of the running surface, tracks provide a ready-made workout, and are a great place for beginning runners to give it a go.

I like track workouts because I like to vary the kinds of running I do. If I do a speed workout or something, it feels more intense on my muscles.
AnneMarie, 32

Most "regulation" tracks are 400 meters around (440 yards), and are shaped like ovals. Run or walk four laps around this track and you've logged one mile. Eight laps . . . two miles, and so on. And because you never feel like you're far away from the beginning (or end) of your run, tracks can make long runs seem short. Most tracks are dotted with all kinds of markers: 10-meter marks, relay baton passing lines, marks for where hurdles should be set up and so on. I usually use only the starting marker and the 200-meter mark (half of a lap) myself. Although sometimes if I'm bored I play a game of "step on a crack" with the various lines on the track, avoiding the horizontal lines at all costs. The downside of track running is that it can be a little monotonous, as each loop only takes a few minutes. Say you're running two miles. That would be eight laps—

enough that you might lose count. But, if you can stand the same scenery loop after loop, the benefits of running on tracks far outweigh the negatives. Hear me out.

Besides easily keeping track of the number of miles or half-miles you've run in any given workout, tracks are great places if you're doing any kind of speed workout or want to figure out what your exact pace is and stick to it. For example, say you want to run one mile in ten minutes. Do the math. Divide ten minutes by four laps, and you find out that it should take you two minutes and thirty seconds (2:30) to finish each lap, "quarter" or "400." If you're wearing a running watch, or even a watch with a second hand, note your starting time, and then check in as you pass your starting spot on lap one. You can then slow down or speed up after the first lap, depending on how you need to adjust your pace to make your goal. Sometimes, if I really need a mind distraction, I'll do math games in my head to pass the time. So if I'm running ten-minute miles, I'll figure out how fast each quarter of a lap should take me, half of a lap and so on. Hey, it makes the laps go by faster . . . what can I say?

I find that I run on tracks the most when I'm traveling, because I "know the course," and I can always find a track close by. A few years before I moved to Los Angeles, I was here on business and stayed with a friend in Santa Monica. My trip was only a few weeks before my first marathon, which I was training for with a lot of trepidation. I'm one of those people that has a hard time running when I'm out of town and my schedule is broken. I am a creature of routine. And with the marathon coming up, I was especially worried about not running enough miles that week. I knew that I wouldn't fare well by setting out on foot from my friend's apartment to face unknown streets, hills and the possibility of getting lost, so I drove to the nearby campus of UCLA. Talk about a nice track! When I was in high school, I used to dream about running on the UCLA track team. I knew I wasn't good enough, but it was nice to dream. But on that day, and for the rest of that week, I *saw* the UCLA track team, and even ran my laps at the same time they were working out. It was actually pretty cool. All of these intense athletes were doing drills, hurdling, jumping, sprinting and I pretended, just for that hour, that I was one of them.

• Go down to the start of the 100-meter dash (the far end of the straightaway). Get down in a starting position, pretend you hear a starting gun and take off! Repeat this several times, running all the way to the other end of the straightaway.

• Run with a friend, and have her start first. When she reaches the halfway mark, you start. Try to keep the distance between the two of you equal as you continue doing your laps.

• Time your first lap. Try to maintain the exact same speed for your next and upcoming laps. See how close you can get.

Check out your local colleges for indoor tracks as well. They can be welcome relief from the cold winter, and many colleges allow people to train indoors for a seasonal fee. Just be aware of track etiquette, as you'll be sharing the track with other runners. Run your slower loops toward the outside lanes of the track—the faster runners and sprinters will usually be taking up the inside lanes. And if you hear someone yelling "track!" behind you, get out of the way! That means someone's coming through faster than you, and you'd better make way for them.

Sidewalks

You might have realized by now that running is my source of peace. My way to stay sane in an otherwise crazy, loud and stressful city. When I left for a late-night run one night, I had no idea that it would be among my best in years. And it all took place on the sidewalk. I had gotten home from work around ten o'clock—too late to do my usual loop in Central Park, but I really needed to "destress" with a run. When I walked out my front door ten minutes later, changed and ready to go, I had no idea where I was going, or for how long. I just started to run.

I like running on the road, because I set out from someplace, and I'd know I have to run back. On a treadmill, it's too easy to push stop. Colleen, 26

Since I couldn't run in the park, I decided to follow along Fifth Avenue and turn around at the Plaza Hotel thirty blocks south for a three-mile run. But when I got to the golden statues marking the Plaza, I wanted more. I was just starting to feel good. So I continued along Central Park South, planning to retrace my route back home in a few minutes. But when I turned around and headed back east, I still wasn't satisfied. So I kept on running. With no planned route in mind, I cut down Sixth Avenue and suddenly found myself in the nighttime of midtown. I started to smile.

I soaked in the sights and energy around me, and ran past the hoards of tourists waiting to squeeze into a booth at Planet Hollywood. I made my way along the fluorescent sign outside Radio City Music Hall, running around the mass exodus of concertgoers spilling out. Cutting up through the tree-lined plaza leading to Rockefeller Center, I spotted the bench where I used to spend my lunch breaks the summer I interned at NBC News.

There were no other runners to be found—only tourists, executives on expense accounts, and homeless people camping out in the doorways of buildings abandoned for the night. But even though I could clearly see all the people around me, I felt as though my own presence was going unnoticed. It was a very strange sensation to feel so invisible and so vibrant at the same time.

Passing the Plaza Hotel for the second time, I headed for home on the cobblestone pathway along the park. Exhausted, I got home a little after eleven o'clock. My run had worked. My stress had dissolved, drummed out of my body with the pounding of my feet along the pavement. If I remember correctly, it took me a while to get to sleep that night. I had a runner's high like I hadn't had in months. Not only was my head clear and focused, but for the first time in years I got back a little of that much-needed energy that drew me to New York in the first place.

> • **Pretend you are a car trying to make all of the green lights.** Speed up if you're approaching a light that is green so you can try to make it through, and slow down if you're approaching a red light. The object is to keep running without having to stop for a light.
>
> • **Play step on a crack.**

Now, I'm not saying that every run on a sidewalk is going to bring you these same kinds of emotional rewards, but I am saying, "Hey, you never know." Yes, the traffic lights can be a pain in the butt to stop for, and noise and fumes from traffic can be annoying as well. But, on the other hand, the nearness of traffic and street lights make sidewalks safe alternatives for late-night runs, or runs anytime at all.

Treadmills

If you're a member of a gym, chances are you've walked or run on a treadmill before, even if just as part of your warm-up. While treadmills aren't my first choice for a run, there are some great aspects to this indoor experience. You may find that running on treadmills brings you the same satisfaction as running outdoors, or more. Like many aspects of running, it's a very personal thing. I know many women who prefer running on a treadmill to the outdoors because they're much more in control of their distance and pacing, and this can be very useful for beginning runners. You can get a good sense of what different mile paces feel like, and be very accurate in measuring the time and distance you've run.

Icy conditions outside usually send me to the treadmill, because worrying about ice takes away from me having a stress-free run.
Emily, 29

Travel tip: Use the plastic laundry bag in your hotel room closet to store your sweaty running clothes in your luggage.

The experience of running on a treadmill is much different than running outdoors on any surface. Treadmills are generally inside of gyms, which amuse and distract their patrons with music, television, movies and mirrors. All of these things can definitely keep a person energized to finish a run—the music to motivate, the television to distract and the mirror to remind you how good you look. But the differences go past the mere running environment. Running on treadmills is a different experience for your body as well. This is mostly because the motion of the treadmill itself assists your body in completing its stride. As

I like the versatility of running on the treadmill, especially living in PA in the winter. If I can't get out with the kids, they can just come down to the basement with me, and I can get a workout in.
Deena, 32

- Try to set the speed for the treadmill so that your feet land with the beat of the music in the background. If a faster song comes on, speed it up. A slow song, bring it down.

- If you're watching television, speed it up during the commercial breaks.

- Some treadmills have "random" settings to spice up your workout with the occasional hill.

the treadmill moves back, it not only forces you to put one foot in front of the other—but it gives you a bit of a push off in the process. This may not make any difference to you if you train on treadmills year round, but if you are a treadmill runner in the winters, you'll find you'll have to go through a bit of an adjustment when you head to the great outdoors in the spring.

I've found that the emotional experience of running on a treadmill is quite different than running outdoors. Generally, my primary goal in running is to unwind, process and feel self-fulfilled. And it's the experience of running outdoors, being part of nature and the elements, that really synthesizes this for me. But don't take my word for it. Try it out. If you're a runner who likes to have a Walkman handy and move to the latest groove, you might find treadmills are a convenient and safe way to run, and that you can always log your miles, rain or shine.

What to Run On

Depending on where you run, the very surface will feel a little different. Here is an idea of what you can expect from the different kinds of running surfaces you might encounter on your journeys.

Tarmac and Cement

If you're a road runner or sidewalk runner, you'll find that tarmac and cement don't "give" much when your feet land on the ground. Running on hard surfaces like these can take some getting used to, and while probably the most common running surface, they're also the ones that place the most wear and tear on your body, although advancements in shoe technology have certainly diminished this effect. If you're running on harder surfaces like these, you may want to make sure you're running in a shoe with supportive cushioning, one that can absorb some of the shock before distributing it to your knees and other joints. A common problem that can result from running on tarmac and cement surfaces is "shin splints." If you've ever experienced a burning sensation along the front or sides of your shin during or after a run, this is probably shin splints. Ice and aspirin can help relieve some of the pain associated with this familiar ailment, but switching to a softer running surface like dirt or grass is your best bet to deal with this problem. For more on shin splints, see chapter Nine.

Dirt and Grass

If I had my druthers, dirt or grass would be the running surface I'd always choose. These surfaces provide enough support that you don't sink too much, but also have an element of shock absorption that your body will appreciate. Be careful if running on dirt or grass while it's raining or when the ground is damp, as grass can be slippery. Wear a shoe with a good sole on it, like a trail running shoe, to prevent slipping and sliding on

I like running on dirt because it feels more cushiony. I run on an old railroad line that's been converted to a trail, with a packed dirt surface.
Michele, 33

grass. Likewise, keep an eye out for any small pebbles or stones in your way to avoid overturning an ankle or tripping.

Track Surfaces

Running on soft track surfaces, whether cinder, rubber or tartan, is great for your body. Cinder tracks are the least desirable, as they can be especially dusty, and the cinders are loose. If you're running fast, you may find that you don't have great traction on the cinders. But look around . . . most likely a high school or college in your area has a rubber track (usually red, orange or green) or tartan track, and after running on this soft, bouncy surface, you'll be sold. The surface of these tracks has a bit of a rough finish to it, giving you enough support that you don't have to worry about sliding, but is smooth enough to give you a nice ride.

I never run on a treadmill. I just like to be outside.
Laura, 36

Treadmills

Running on treadmills provides a comfortable enough experience that you shouldn't have to worry about things like shin splints or other aches and pains. Generally, these have soft rubber surfaces that give back enough of a bounce to counter those ailments. However, at the same time, treadmills can be difficult to adjust to, and you may find yourself having to concentrate on your every step to avoid going too far to either side (I know I do).

Sand

You know those movies where the heroine goes for a beautiful, romantic jog along the beach? Don't get swept up in the Hol-

lywoodization of exercise. Running on sand is a tricky proposi-
tion, and is hard on your calves and feet to boot. If you've tried it
before, you know what I mean. As you try to push off with your
back foot, you'll find that it sinks into the sand, making your calf
muscle do extra work to keep you moving forward. For these
same reasons, running on loose sand can be a great leg-
strengthening workout. Just be aware of what you're in store for.
The damp, packed sand close to the water's edge is a more stable
surface. If you choose to run on the beach, take my advice, and
don't do it barefoot. You may end up straining a foot muscle. Put
on some supportive shoes, and go toward the water's edge.

I love running on sand. Occasionally I dune climb on the soft sand, which is one of the best exercises on the planet, but it's really hard.
Libby, 41

Summary

So, what's it gonna be? The local park or a run through the
woods on a winding trail? Or maybe a few laps on the local
track. Whatever your choice, just remember that you have lots
of options, and I encourage you to explore them all and vary
your runs. Spicing up your running life with new courses is a
surefire way to stave off boredom and open yourself to whatever is waiting for you. Maybe you'll have a night run like the
one I had in Manhattan. Or maybe you'll find a path that takes
you past a historic landmark . . . you've lived there all these
years, and you never even knew it was there. I guarantee
you . . . every fresh running place will give you the chance to
discover something new. Just keep your eyes open and find it.

7.

To Carb or Not to Carb:

Eating to Run

The year I ran my first marathon, the coach of my running club gave me some training suggestions to get ready for the race. And I use the word *race* liberally, for the marathon for me is more aptly described as a test of will, but nothing like a race. Perhaps my favorite part of training for this first marathon was his prescribed diet for the seven days before the big event. "Eat as much junk as you want," Jorge said. And by junk he meant fatty, calorie-laden food—ice cream, potato chips, French fries, the works. I didn't question his advice. In fact, I followed it vigorously. And what do you know . . . it worked. Although I had only decided to run the marathon two months earlier, I finished the run in a respectable four hours and 59 minutes. And I managed to run the entire thing. During that week, as I indulged my every food craving, I managed to build up enough stored "energy" to keep me going all the way through those 26.2 miles. And while his advice might have been unconventional, it worked for me.

Now that I've been through the marathon process a few more times, I don't follow that same exact diet regimen. But my experience as described above does prove that there's more than one way to eat to run. Let me preface this chapter by saying that I am not a nutritionist. But I've done some homework, and this chapter combines research along with personal experience.

I don't really believe in the word diet. I think it has a negative connotation and can drive people crazy. My basic philosophy is everything in moderation.
Emily, 29

Carbohydrates, Fat and Protein

There are countless schools of thought regarding diet and nutrition for runners and non runners alike. Most of the debate revolves around the ratio of carbohydrates, fat and protein in your diet. For years and years, the traditional thinking has been that most people, specifically runners, are best served by high carbohydrate, low fat diets. In fact, many nutritionists and trainers still go by this theory. But in the last ten years or so, some new perspectives have emerged that have challenged this notion, most notably the now infamous Atkins Diet, which is based on all fat and protein with little or no carbohydrates, and the Zone diet, which uses the model of a diet consisting of forty percent carbohydrates, thirty percent fat and thirty percent protein. Both of these diets and their founders have developed a large following. I'm sure you know people who go out to lunch and order a bacon cheeseburger with no bun and a side of sausage in strict adherence to the Atkins diet. Or maybe you've done it yourself.

Although I'm guilty of experimenting with my fair share of fad diets over the years, I've never tried the Atkins diet. I did buy *The Zone,* and tend to think that the ideas behind it are

I'm pretty poor at diet management, but I am aware of trying to eat proteins at times, and balancing that out. I think I eat more carbs than I need to.
Emily, 30

pretty solid. But what I've found works best for my body is to maintain a *balance* in my diet. Our bodies need a little bit of everything—not too much, not too little. And that includes fats and carbohydrates. But do runners have special dietary needs? Here's a look at the big three food types and how they play a role in the runner's diet.

Carbohydrates in a Runner's Diet

Since I'm currently training for a marathon, carbohydrates are making up a larger part of my diet than they normally might. There is no doubt about it. Carbohydrates equal fuel for runners in many ways. If I've got a long training run on a Sunday morning, I'll make sure I eat a bowl of pasta or have a lot of rice or bread Saturday night. Simple carbohydrates like bread, rice and pasta are easily accessible as a form of energy, and this comes in handy around mile fourteen or so—when your body is looking for anything it's got to keep it going. The problem with high carbohydrate diets in general is that if you're not doing long bouts of exercise, whatever carbohydrates your body doesn't use settles in your fat cells, ultimately becoming fat. You might find that if you're eating a lot of carbohydrates and not doing a lot of cardiovascular exercise, your body feels bloated. And if you're doing only moderate amounts of exercise, according to Dr. Philip Maffetone in the *Washington Running Report*, 40 percent of the carbohydrates you ingest aren't immediately used up and instead add to your fat stores.

A good thing to keep in mind is that as the intensity and duration of your workouts increase, so should your carbohydrate intake. So, while carbohydrates are absolutely an important part of our diet, the old school of thought recommending the bulk of our food come from simple and complex carbohydrates may not work best for your body, especially if one of your goals in running is to reduce body fat.

Fat in a Runner's Diet

Many of us think of fat as the enemy, and opt for fat-free foods that might be higher in carbohydrates and calories instead. I used to be very antifat, and like many other women, thought if I stuck to eating fat-free foods, the weight would just melt off of me. Well, the fat-free era appears to be over, and the truth about such snacks is now known. In many cases, fat-free foods are high in calories and carbohydrates, and we know what happens to unused carbohydrates in our body, right? I advocate moderate amounts of fat in our diets. Again, in keeping with the goal of a balanced diet, to eliminate fat completely would be a bad thing. The truth is, a little fat in your diet is a good thing.

There are three kinds of fat that you're probably already aware of: saturated fat, polyunsaturated fat and monounsaturated fat. Saturated fat is the kind we should try to limit, as it's responsible for raising "bad" cholesterol (LDLs) and is linked closely to heart disease. Saturated fat comes mainly from animal products, like butter, cheese, meat, as well as oil (coconut oil is especially high). It is recommended that our diet consist of very little saturated fat—approximately ten percent of our total daily calories. Unsaturated fats, on the other hand, can actually be good for you, as they can help to raise levels of "good cholesterol" (HDLs),

I monitor my fat. I eat about 65 grams a day, and I try to stick to that. I often have to make a conscious effort to get enough fat in my diet.
Michele, 33

which can counter the effects of bad cholesterol in your body. Polyunsaturated and monounsaturated fats can be found in things like peanut oil, olives and soy. So, do the standard rules regarding fat intake apply to runners, too? Dr. Kamal Jabbour, a runner and columnist for the *Syracuse Post-Standard* wrote in 1999 that it is important for runners to eat fatty foods. He refers to a study at the University of Buffalo that determined "runners who limit their fat intake compromise their immune system and increase their risk of infections and disease." According to earlier studies at the University of Buffalo, competitive runners with moderate-to-high fat diets increased their endurance without increasing their weight, blood pressure, heart rate or cholesterol.

TYPE OF FAT	DESCRIPTION
Saturated	Stimulates production of LDL ("bad" cholesterol). *Animal fats (meat, poultry, dairy), fast foods, palm oil, coconut oil, butter*
Polyunsaturated	Lowers LDL ("bad" cholesterol) levels, but lowers HDL ("good" cholesterol) levels as well. *Sunflower oil, soybean oil, corn oil, fish oils*
Monounsaturated	Lowers LDL ("bad" cholesterol) levels while leaving HDL ("good" cholesterol) levels alone. *Olive oil, canola oil, peanut oil, avocado*

Protein in a Runner's Diet

When I think of protein, I tend to picture those protein shakes and powder mixes sold at health food stores. The ones that promise bulky muscles on men and defined strong muscles for women. My ex-boyfriend used to drink protein mixes with the hope it would make him bulk up, and it did, but he

For a while I was a vegetarian and I wasn't doing a good job of monitoring my protein intake, and one day after running I had decided to have some meat, and the rest of the day, I felt really good and I wasn't tired. It was then I realized I wasn't getting enough protein in my diet.
Bridget, 32

also just got big in general as a result. But that's another story. Beyond the benefits it provides in terms of building up muscle mass, protein is also key in repairing muscle damage that can be caused by exercises like running.

According to Dr. Liz Applegate, nutrition columnist and editor of *Runner's World* magazine, eating more protein could improve not only your running, but also your overall health. In an article she wrote for *Runner's World* entitled "Protein Primer," she explains that too little protein in your diet can affect overall health, and our bodies' won't heal injuries or illnesses as effectively. People who run regularly use up more protein in a day, and therefore they have higher protein needs than people who aren't habitual exercisers.

IRON AND CALCIUM: WOMEN'S SPECIAL NEEDS

Women need higher levels of iron and calcium in their diets because of menstruation and osteoporosis. Good sources of calcium include: dairy, leafy green vegetables, salmon. Good sources of iron include: cream of wheat, beef and spinach.

So where do you get protein in your diet? Protein comes from plants and animals—meats like fish and chicken are chock full of protein. For vegetarians, tofu and soy are excellent sources of protein, as are dairy products like milk, eggs and cheese. Be aware though, that many forms of protein are also high in fat (like cheese), so choosing your protein from lower fat sources like fish and tofu probably makes more sense.

The Importance of Water for Women and Runners

About four years ago, I had my body fat calculations done by Michael Youseff, an aerobics instructor at my gym. I'll keep the results to myself if you don't mind, but one thing that Michael said was that my hydration levels were really low, and that this could affect my body fat reading. I was surprised to hear that I was dehydrated, because I drank a fair amount of fluids throughout the day. Michael challenged me to start drinking at least sixty-four ounces of water every day (about two one-liter bottles), and he predicted my body fat reading would be more accurate (and more favorable) a month down the road. I accepted his challenge, and true to his prediction, my hydration levels read normal and my body fat calculations were more in line with what I would have expected based on my diet and the amount of exercise I was doing at the time.

We've all read the reports about water and how important it is to maintaining efficiency in our brains and bodies. Water helps our bodies digest food, keeps our skin healthy, helps encourage weight loss by suppressing appetites, flushes the system of toxins, reduces water retention by encouraging the kidneys to work properly, reduces fat deposits in the body, reduces sodium buildup in the body and on and on. So

WATER CAN AND WILL:

- Improve your complexion
- Improve your circulation
- Improve your digestion
- Encourage weight loss
- Suppress your appetite
- Keep you sharp and alert

why are we still so reluctant to drink the recommended amount of water every day? Our bodies are nearly two-thirds water, so it's obviously crucial to our survival and nourishment.

For runners, water is even more important to include in our diet. Reason one is that you need to replace the fluids you sweat out when you exercise, so runners should drink above and beyond the minimum daily recommended amount. Likewise, lean muscle tissue—the kind of tissue that running builds up—is made of more water than other types of muscle tissue, so this again requires that you ingest extra amounts throughout the day.

A good way to make sure you're drinking enough fluids is to monitor the color of your urine. The goal is to be peeing relatively clearly by the afternoon, unless you've just taken some vitamins or medication that might alter the color. Your water intake doesn't have to be comprised only of pure water. Juice, tea and fluid replacement drinks like Gatorade all have high amounts of water in them, as do certain fruits like cantaloupe, oranges, watermelon and so on. Beverages that don't count as water substitutes would be sodas (other than seltzer water) and especially those beverages with caffeine, coffee and alcohol. Alcohol and beverages with caffeine actually serve to dehydrate your body, threatening to undo all of the good you've been doing by drinking water all day.

The good news is, you can never drink too much water—the only possible side effect is that you may find yourself having to go to the bathroom every hour, which can be disruptive if you're in meetings, at work or at a movie. But take comfort—if you're just starting to up your water intake for the first time, your body will begin to get used to your new schedule, and

I recently read that 75 percent of Americans are chronically dehydrated, and I believe it. I drink tons of water.
Eileen, 26

I have recently started to drink even more water and it's making me feel so good. Now I actually crave it.
Alice, 34

eventually you won't have to go to the bathroom quite as frequently.

How Caffeine Affects Running

Caffeine is a wonder drug to many, myself included. I'm not a
coffee drinker. Rather, my preferred method of caffeine intake is
good old-fashioned diet Coke. Stop by my office at nine in the
morning, and you'll catch me eating a breakfast bar and chug-
ging a cold mug of diet Coke. I know I just talked about the
dehydration effects of caffeine—diet Coke is my weakness. This
always shocks people and they are surprised that I would dare
drink something cold and carbonated in the morning as
opposed to hot, bitter coffee. Regardless of your source, I'm sure
at some time or another you've enjoyed the perks of some caffeine in your system. If you're like my husband, caffeine in the
form of coffee and soda is a way of life. Derin can drink a double
espresso at twelve midnight and still be asleep a half-hour later.

Derin also likes to drink coffee before road races, something
that I always found surprising, I guess because coffee gives me
stomach cramps. But after researching the idea of running and
caffeine, I found that many running authorities consider a prerace cup of coffee to be absolutely okay, and that it may even
have benefits for the runner. According to Susan Glen, M.Sc.
Nutrition, at the *Running Room*, caffeine can be beneficial in
endurance runs by fending off fatigue and keeping your muscles' glycogen stores full (this keeps muscles fresh and delays
the onslaught of muscle fatigue in very long runs).

I am incredibly caffeine sensitive, so I rarely even take any in.
Libby, 42

However, all of the effects that caffeine has on your body when you're not running are also true for when you are, like the fact that caffeine acts as a diuretic in your body, and this can lead to dehydration. Also, for many, strong caffeine drinks like coffee result in painful stomach cramps.

Of the different power drinks and gels on the market for runners and other exercisers, many contain caffeine. Those that don't generally mention this on the packaging to let the user know they won't be getting that extra boost. So if you do want to try using caffeine during a race or long run, you may want to try it in the form of a power gel and see how it works for you.

Energy Bars and Other Enhancement Products

Energy bars and protein bars are hugely popular right now, launched in part by the introduction of the PowerBar to the market in 1987. Since then, all kinds of products have cropped up that are meant to give the athlete extra energy in a pure form of carbohydrate, and many are also being used as meal replacements. For runners, they are best utilized when running distances over ten miles at a time. Here's a look at the more popular energy and enhancement products on the market.

Energy Bars

Most energy bars have an average of 250 calories, and are full of potassium, carbohydrates and protein. I generally eat

I usually don't use sports drinks but I do use GU or a piece of a Clif Bar when I'm doing more than a ten-mile run. I have one of those waist belts that has room for other things so I always have a snack with me.
Sarah, 28

these the morning of a long run or race as a breakfast substitute. I used to eat these while I was running for a boost, but with the introduction of PowerGels and GU, which are more portable and easier to open when on the run, I find I'm not eating so many bars anymore. The more popular energy bars on the market include:

- *Clif Bars:* Very high in carbohydrates, this bar is made using all-natural ingredients and comes in ten unusual flavors like Apricot and Carrot Cake.

- *Harvest Bars:* Created by the folks at PowerBar, these low-fat energy bars are made with natural ingredients and sweetened with brown rice syrup instead of sugar.

- *Luna Bars:* Dubbed as the "whole nutrition bar for women," Luna Bars are made from the manufacturers of Clif Bars and have soy protein at the top of their ingredients list. They're also high in calcium and other recommended vitamins for women.

- *PowerBar:* Undoubtedly the number-one energy bar, this is a low-fat, high-nutrient energy bar. These can be difficult to open, especially if you want to eat it midrun. Many runners prepare these by cutting them into bite-sized slices beforehand so they can easily eat them while running.

- *PR Ironman Triathlon Bar:* These bars subscribe to the theory outlined in the popular book *The Zone,* which recommends a 40/30/30 ratio in your diet (40 percent calories from carbohydrates, 30 percent from protein and 30 percent from fat). These are designed to help the eater burn stored body fat for energy when you are exercising instead of tapping into the readily available carbohydrates.

Gels

More recently, gels have come on the market as a substitute for energy bars for athletes in the midst of performing. It's kind of hard to munch down a PowerBar when you're trying to run a long distance, although I've done it many times before. But bars can be heavy and awkward to carry, harder to open up while running, and present difficulties when chewing and swallowing while running. Hence, the introduction of the performance gel—a liquid gel energy boost easily toted, easily opened and easily ingested.

- *GU:* Yes, this product is really called GU (pronounced "goo"). And it's really yummy to boot. GU is nicknamed "Fast Food for Athletes," although I still think of a Wendy's Jr. Cheeseburger Deluxe when I think of fast food. Mmm. GU is designed to give the user quick and efficient energy, without all of the fiber, protein and fat that many energy bars have. GU's are, simply put, simple carbohydrate calories, and they'll give you an instant boost. They're best ingested by sucking the "gu" out of the small plastic pouch and washing it down with a mouthful of water. These are the gels I use when training for the marathon—my rule is a packet of GU every six miles or so. GU comes in a half-dozen flavors.

I always take PowerGels when I'm training for marathons. They're very digestible and they give me the carbs I need. I use that, and OJ in a water bottle.
Gail, 52

I think I need to refuel more often than most people do. During the marathon I ate a PowerGel every six miles, and if I didn't, I started to feel light-headed and shaky. But as soon as I ate one, I was okay.
Christie, 29

- **PowerGels:** Made by the makers of PowerBar, PowerGels are the other popular performance gel on the market. PowerGels are a "concentrated carbohydrate gel that delivers immediate energy during intense athletic activity." Like GU, they come in caffeinated or noncaffeinated flavors. I have used PowerGels in the past, and they're quite yummy (I'm partial to the mixed berry blend), although I have found that they go through me a little too quickly (if you know what I mean), and I have found myself in search of a bathroom a few miles after ingesting one.

Fluid Replacement Drinks

Gatorade is the forefather (or foremother) of fluid replacement drinks, and is still among the most popular drinks to replace electrolytes in the body. But today, Gatorade has some competition in the runner's market.

- **Cytomax:** Cytomax is my fluid replacement drink of choice. It was recommended to us by our neighbors Tip and Bridget who used it while running the LA Marathon last year. A few months ago, I picked up a container of Cytomax at a sporting goods store near work, and Derin and I tested it out during a run. It was an easily digestible, tasty drink that kept us energized throughout our entire run. Self-described as the "world's most scientifically advanced complex carbohydrate, electrolyte performance energy drink," Cytomax helps the runner stay hydrated, maintain energy and not get fatigued during long workouts. Cytomax comes as a powder and is mixed with water and ingested periodically throughout extended runs.

- **Gatorade:** Gatorade has been around since 1967, when researchers at the University of Florida (their mascot, the Gators) developed the drink to help the school's football players stay hydrated and quickly replace the fluids and sugars that the athletes were losing in intensely hot conditions. Today, Gatorade is arguably the most popular sports drink on the market. Its primary goal is to replace the electrolytes that are lost in your body when you become dehydrated. In fact, Gatorade has many of the same ingredients as something called ORT (oral rehydration therapy), which is a solution used in the developing world to help prevent children with diarrhea from dying of dehydration.

- **ProLyte:** ProLyte contains simple and complex carbohydrates, vitamins, electrolytes and 30 milligrams of pure caffeine. Its goal is to help keep your body running its most efficient without fatiguing, and keep you hydrated at the same time.

- **Ultima:** I have recently gotten familiar with Ultima because it's the official sports drink of the LA Marathon, and I tried it last week for the first time during a long training run. And I have to say, it did my body good. Ultima was designed specifically to rehydrate the body, and doesn't have as many simple sugars as some of the other drinks on the market. Rather, it is comprised of large amounts of potassium, along with calcium and magnesium, which

I generally drink water on my long runs, unless it's an organized race. Then I'll drink Gatorade. Emily, 30

according to Ultima, "protects the muscles from cramping and enhances neuromuscular performance." Ultima is best used by runners going out for longer distances, who need some help in the endurance department. It generally comes as a powder mix, which should be combined with water.

When to Eat in Relation to Your Runs

I remember as a kid being sternly warned about the dangers of swimming after eating. I was told you could get stomach cramps that were so painful you'd drown. Boy, did my vivid imagination go to town with that bit of information. Well, while there are no threats of drowning here, I do generally run on an empty stomach or after a light meal, and it's best to wait until about an hour after eating before going out for a run.

Morning Runs

If I run during the week and it's not too lengthy (under five miles), I usually do the run without eating first, and only drinking a glass of water or some juice. I'll tend to eat a bowl of cereal and a piece of fruit once my run is over. However, if I'm running a long run on the weekend (anything over six miles), I'll eat something light first, like a Nutri-Grain Bar or a Harvest Bar. My running partner Christie has to eat something before her morning runs or else her stomach will be growling and panging the whole way.

Afternoon or Late Day Runs

If I'm running after work, I'll generally try to eat a piece of fruit as a late afternoon snack to give me energy and tide me over until dinner. But I also pay attention to what I'm eating for lunch. If I know a run is in the cards for later that day, I'll skip the meatball special at IKEA (complete with gravy and new potatoes . . . mmm). Lighter, simpler foods will ensure that my body doesn't waste all its energy digesting lunch, and save a little for my evening run.

Most importantly, *listen to your body*. Like, many other aspects of running, how you should eat to best fuel your body and your run is a very personal choice. Use trial and error to find out whether or not stocking up on carbohydrates makes a difference as you tag on miles. Try some of the enhancement products and see if you feel the energy boost they are supposed to provide. But be smart. Eat sensibly and keep a balance.

8

Keeping the Faith:

How to Stay Motivated

About one month after running my first marathon, I signed up for a local 10K (6.2 miles) race. I hadn't run in exactly four weeks, and was really looking forward to getting back into a routine. Even though I'm not a big fan of the 10K racing distance (a 2–3 mile race is my ideal), I thought that after running 26.2 miles, this considerably shorter race would be a walk in the park for me. Well, it was. Literally. About three miles into the race, I felt a sharp pain on the outside of my right knee. I slowed down to a walk, and was embarrassed when the race officials asked me if I was okay. I smiled, answered "yes," and started to run again. A half-mile later, I stopped in pain again, this time opting to just walk home. I had never dropped out of a race before. I was really bummed out and disappointed in myself.

Well, reality set in. This was only the first time of many in recent memory when a run wouldn't feel so great, and I would lose the desire to keep on going, let alone go out for a run in the

Running didn't become part of my lifestyle overnight. But for me, I need exercise to maintain stability in my life, and running does that for me.
Emily, 29

first place. This used to get me down, and I would find myself questioning my commitment as a runner, and whether or not I even had the right to call myself a runner. But over the years, I've learned that this feeling is just part of being human, part of being a runner, part of being a woman. And one day or one week of lethargy doesn't mean it's all over. Every day that you get out there and run is a day that you're doing something positive for yourself. I've found that the best way to maintain the enthusiasm most people experience during the first few weeks of a new regimen is to dig deep and create a foolproof plan to keep yourself going.

A few years ago, I took my dog, Ari, to the dog run down by Gracie Mansion in Carl Schurz Park (in New York City), and I saw this girl jogging around a very small courtyard. She had her Walkman in hand, and was just going around and around. And I thought to myself, "How can she possibly be getting any enjoyment out of that?" It looked so boring. I got dizzy just watching her.

News flash. The bare naked truth is . . . running is sometimes boring. There. I've said it. But hey. Think about all of those things we really enjoy doing that get boring sometimes. Going to the movies. Going to work. But that doesn't mean that we don't do them anymore. We just find ways to make them more stimulating. For example, a full tub of popcorn, large diet Coke and a package of Twizzlers can make even the most boring movie an enjoyable experience. My point is, more likely than not, you'll have runs where you'll be anticipating the end.

And boredom is just one of the things you'll be up against as you embark on this new running lifestyle. There's work. The

When you have two kids you have to really want to do it to make the time to get out there and run. It's hard at times, but it's a priority in my life. So I make the time.
Deena, 32

holidays. PMS. Rain. Snow. Achy muscles. Television. Family. Friends. I mean, how could someone possibly manage to run when they're contending with PMS, a ton of last-minute Christmas shopping, snow, preparation for a family visit and a frantic work deadline? There's no easy answer. I personally use a whole slew of different methods to keep myself running, because inevitably, keeping my running date with myself during busy times like these helps me focus more clearly on what has to be done. It gives me the sense that I have some control over my destiny during a time when I otherwise feel that I'm a pinball being bounced around an arcade game. Plainly put, it keeps me sane.

Depending on what's going on in my life, running can be either a large or small burden. But it's always just as rewarding. Sometimes the more challenging it is to squeeze in a run, the better it will be. The harder it is to scrape my body off of my bed at 6:45 in the morning, the better I'll feel when I'm through with my run. I do go through phases—usually when I'm on a higher mileage running schedule—when I get addicted to running. I notice this more on days when I don't run—I feel as though I'm going through a sort of withdrawal. But even when I'm in this frame of mind, it's always as a result of some sort of motivational strategy I've been using to keep myself running.

Sometimes I have to devise methods for just putting on my running shoes and walking out the front door. I have to believe that this is the case for any runner who isn't training and competing at an elite level. We're not going to be winning any medals here, so we need more motivation. Here are some of my tricks of the trade. I hope you find a few that work for you!

Make (and Keep) Running Dates

If you're like most women, you've got a hectic schedule. A job, outside interests, a social life, a personal life. I definitely have a hard time fitting it all in. And more often than not, it's the exercise—that time we've set aside to do something so positive and healthy for ourselves—that gets sacrificed. About five years ago, I started making running dates with friends. For a solid year, I ran in New York with a close friend of mine, Frank. We had both recently gone through pretty horrible breakups (read: we were both dumped by our significant others), and we started running together as a way to do something good for ourselves when we were otherwise feeling so bad, and to have a solid chunk of commiseration a few times a week. It worked out well for both of us. As we ran, I would go through what my therapist said earlier in the week—free therapy for Frank, and I would feel strengthened by talking about what I was learning. As you might imagine, the runs flew by. And I looked forward to them. We both did.

I tell everyone that running is the best therapy for the cheapest price. It's mindless how great it is.

Sue, 55

But what if you haven't just been dumped? Well, then. Make running dates anyway! A few months ago, I made the switch from running in the evenings to the mornings— something I never thought I'd do. But a friend of mine down the street runs religiously in

- **Put up a sign at work to see if there are any runners in your company you could schedule runs with.**

- **Join a local running club—they often have bulletin boards to help people find running partners.**

- **Try making a running date even once a week! Set distance or time goals with your partner. This will help your running even on days you're doing it alone!**

the mornings, and one day I decided to try it out. Kind of like a test run. We agreed I'd ease into it. First one morning a week. Then a week later, two mornings. And so on. It only took two morning runs with Christie and I was hooked. We talk about everything. Or sometimes we don't talk at all. It works like this. My alarm goes off at 6:45. I am extremely tired. And cold. My down comforter is *very warm*. I hit snooze. 6:55. I remember that Christie is going to be sitting on her front porch one block away at 7:15, and without any further thought, I flip back the covers and trek down the hall to the bathroom. By the time I've brushed my teeth, I'm awake. I throw on some clothes, grab my keys, and step out the door. I cross the street between Christie's and my house, and I see her pop her head up from behind the bushes by her steps. She stands up and waves at me with both hands and grins sleepily, and I do the same. Next thing I know, my run is over. Relatively painless.

Vary the Route

A change of scenery always does the body good. If you live in a city like New York, you may feel that your running options are limited. But, with a little creativity and asking other runners about their routes, you might discover variety and new challenges in your town. In New York, I had a few routes that I stuck to for the most part. But even reversing the direction of a running loop adds its own challenges, including hills in different places.

If I was heading out for my run unusually late, sometimes I would alter my routine and run along the outside of the park or somewhere more populated and well-lit. Sometimes I run on tracks not because I'm in the mood for a speed workout or anything, but on nights when I'm really tired, running on a track feels more manageable. That way if I run out of steam I won't find myself stuck three miles from home. Sometimes just heading out the door without any set course in mind can be a reward in itself. Following your feet can bring new sights, sounds and stimuli to your run. That night run I had in Manhattan, now four years ago, is still so vivid to me.

Changing my running route is very important because I run for noncompetitive reasons. So, while I'm running what keeps me motivated is what I'm visually experiencing.
AnneMarie, 32

Now that I'm in Los Angeles, I feel that my running options are wide open. In the year since I've been here I've run on the sidewalks and streets in my neighborhood in West Hollywood, along the paved path that lines the beach in Santa Monica and Venice, through the canyons (and steep hills, ugh) of the Malibu Mountains, and around Lake Hollywood under the shadow of

- **Do a run where you make up the route as you go along—just make sure you're familiar with the neighborhood so you don't get lost!**

- **Plan a day trip to a state park with a friend or partner—pack a picnic and change of clothes for some dining and hiking after your run.**

- **Run your standard run in the reverse direction . . . notice how different the view is from your new vantage point.**

the Hollywood sign. Sometimes Derin and I make our weekend runs into true outings . . . we'll plan a day at the beach, and start it off with a run.

Changing your running route is a great way to explore new areas, too. I know that's easy for me to say, considering I just moved here a year ago and everything is still pretty new to me. But I bet you'll find that even if you've lived somewhere your whole life there are running paths, parks and trails you never knew existed.

One last note—varying your running route is also important for reasons of safety. The Road Runners Club of America (RRCA) recommends that runners change their routines fairly often so that your schedule and routes don't become too familiar to anyone you wouldn't want them to (more on this in the next chapter).

Brunch

I include the idea of brunch in this chapter because, to be honest, it's a pretty big motivational tool for me. And for a few of my friends. Barely a weekend goes by where a morning run isn't followed by a hefty and fulfilling dining experience at one of the local restaurants. Ah . . . brunch. My favorite meal of the week. The longer the run, the more I feel I can indulge in pancakes, waffles, omelets or French toast. Or sometimes all of the above.

On the weekends we go to a nice spot, usually the beach, and go for a nice long run, and go to a different restaurant and have a big brunch. It makes the whole day a lot more fun.
Bridget, 32

In New York, these brunches were with Derin and Frank. The run? Frankly, it was just a precursor to a great meal at Jackson Hole on 92nd and Madison. But we ran, and that was the important thing. Besides brunch, of course. When my husband and I went back to New York for a long weekend visit last August, I planned to do my four-mile loop in Central Park on Saturday morning. I missed Central Park so much, and couldn't wait to be back in its embrace. I invited Frank to join us for the run for old times' sake. I told my two girlfriends of our plan, and they opted to join us. I dubbed it the *First Annual Debbie*

Reber Central Park Run. In the end there were six of us, six people who'd never run together before—all different paces, different running styles, different methods for getting through runs. It was pretty funny to me at the time—this ragamuffin group joined together for a run. But it was the whole experience—the togetherness, the run, the company and the orange juice, toast and two eggs scrambled—that was so great. I loved it. And I hope we do it every time I go back.

Now that we're in sunny Southern California, we've taken to running with our next-door neighbors, who just happen to be marathon runners. A couple of times a month, we do a race together (I use the word *together* loosely, as Tip and Bridget kick both of our asses when it comes to speed) or a long run at the beach, and then go out for breakfast. We often spend a chunk of our run talking about what we're going to order for breakfast or where we should eat. I've finished races visualizing French toast. This has also given Derin and I the opportunity to try out new restaurants. And there are a lot of them in LA, so I don't see this method running dry for quite a while.

> • **Plan a morning run with a friend and pick a restaurant to grab a bite to eat afterwards.**
>
> • **Run in your neighborhood and treat yourself to a home-cooked breakfast—make some French toast or how about some waffles?**

Run with Music

Running with music is definitely a matter of personal preference. For years I used to run with a portable radio, the kind that was extremely light and just strapped on to my running shorts or around my bicep. I listened to, well, this is kind of embarrassing. My station of choice was Lite 106.7 FM—"Love songs from the '70s, '80s and '90s." I liked running with the radio, because of the element of surprise. One time my little radio got me through the hardest part of my run. There's this hill in Central Park called Cat Hill, called such because of an iron statue of a mountain lion that is perched along the grassy hill near the top. This hill is a sprinter's hill—short and steep. At the end of a four-mile run it can be a little daunting. One time I was running, my legs feeling like lead, my body exhausted, my fingers and nose cold from the wind, and I rounded the corner before Cat Hill. Just as the incline began, Donna Summer's "She Works Hard for the Money," a song that I had learned a jazz dance routine to as a 12-year-old, came on the radio. I grinned to myself and pumped up the volume, picking up my pace to a (near) sprint and keeping my feet moving in time with the beat. I can honestly say, Donna got me through the rest of that run. And I thank her for it.

As a matter of safety, running with headphones can be dangerous, especially at night. I know of one woman who stopped running outdoors because she was almost hit by a car two times while crossing streets during her run. She was so caught up in the music she found she wasn't paying attention to what was going on around her. Running with music after dark is dangerous, as you might be considered easy prey for someone who means to do you harm. In fact, the RRCA highly recommends that women never run with music unless it's indoors—it just makes us too vulnerable. Personally, I've been running without any music for the past four or five years. I stopped the first winter I ran outdoors in the evenings because of the safety factor. I found that the overall experience was much more enjoyable after a while. I process things better without music. This is the opposite for some people. So whatever it takes, the soundtrack to *Fame*, Van Halen (my girlfriend AnneMarie's favorite), New Age or whatever, if it makes the run more enjoyable, go for it. Use your best judgment. If you're in an environment where running with music could potentially put you in harm's way, leave the music behind.

Start a Running Log

Being accountable to anything can keep you on the straight and narrow, and I've found that keeping a running log truly works to keep me going. I've been keeping a running log in some form for years. For a while there I was just marking in my calendar the number of miles run on each day in red ink. Then at the bottom right-hand corner of each week I would total up the miles and write them in bold black pen, highlighted in yellow. (Yes, I color code my files at work, too. It's one of my "things.") After that came the Palm Pilot. I started using my stylus to keep track of miles electronically. Very 1990s of me. What I've been doing for the past two years now has worked out the best. I made this chart on my computer (I'm known as the "chart queen" among my colleagues). It's simple enough, but it gives a structure to keep track of my runs, races, mile times, weekly and monthly totals and even when I started running in a new pair of shoes. Now that I've been keeping this chart for so long, I feel as though any serious breaks in running will be glaringly obvious to

I kept a running log for both marathons and I felt it was critically important. I found it reassuring to look back and see that, yes, I had in fact run the miles I needed to prepare.
Gail, 52

anyone who would review the chart. And to me. And to the chart itself. Here's a sample from my training log:

MONTHLY TOTAL MILEAGE		77.5	
New Running Shoes Here . . .			
February 4	Tuesday	5	
	Wednesday	5	
	Friday	3.5	
	Sunday	18.6	3:19:00
Weekly Total Mileage		**32.1**	

I keep a detailed log of my exercise. It helps me to go back and see patterns of when I have more energy, and when I don't. Now I don't beat myself up as much when I don't.
Michele, 33

My running chart has been a great historical record for me, too. I can see how fast I ran certain distances in the past, or see which months I tend to run the most miles. On the same note, I can see where my most difficult running stretches come into play. It's like a living document that I am accountable to. I guess it's similar to when you're dieting and you're supposed to write down everything that you eat over the course of a week to get a better handle on what you're ingesting. One tends to eat better than they normally would during these weeks. Who wants to admit on paper that you had a Krispy Kreme doughnut (let alone two) during your breakfast meeting?

Some people keep running logs in which they write down all kinds of information in addition to the number of miles run. If you have the time, you might find it works for you to keep track of how your runs feel, both physically and emotionally. Was the run hard for you to finish? Did you feel like you could have kept on going? Was the run fulfilling from a mental and emotional point of view? These are really interesting things to note, as you may find some patterns in your own life that relate to your running. For example, maybe on really stressful days, you find that your runs go by quicker and you feel stronger physically. Or perhaps you'll note that on runs during your period, your cramps aren't as intense as when you're not exercising. Our bodies and mind react differently to running, and keeping a detailed running diary can help you get to know your body, through running, a little better. Here are some suggestions for the kinds of things you could keep track of in your running log:

- The distance you ran
- The amount of time you ran
- The course you ran
- What you wore
- What the weather was like
- Whether you ran alone or with someone
- What time of day you ran
- How your run felt
- Other things going on in your life
- How the run fits into your running goals

Sign up for Races

More than any other method, signing up for road races has kept me in running shorts. You may not be interested in running races, or perhaps the idea of a competition is intimidating to you. I completely understand this, and believe me, you are not alone. I do not run road races to win. Or to place in the top ten for that matter. And frankly, I never win or place in the top ten. I do, however, run road races to keep myself going. Road

For me, there is no such thing as not finishing. If you have to walk, you walk. You can always get through it.
Janet, 51

races take place all across the country and fairly frequently. I'd bargain that you could find a road race at least once a month in most counties. So every couple of months I'll do a search for road races in the area, and then sign up for them, one by one, by fax or e-mail. Ten to twenty dollars a pop. And *ta-da*. I've just ensured myself another month or two of running. I know that technically I don't have to run the race just because I signed up for it, but then I'd be throwing money away, and that's not a good thing. That's like signing up for a gym membership, having the money automatically deducted from your savings account and then never showing up. I've done that, too. But for some reason, signing up for a race, and knowing that my commemorative size medium t-shirt and numbered bib is waiting to be picked up and worn, compels me to show up. And if I'm going to show up, I'd better at least know that I'm going to be able to run the distance. Running races also invariably helps you with your own personal record or PR, as you'll undoubtedly find yourself running races faster than your normal runs, if for no other reason than an extra boost of adrenaline.

> Run for a cause! Many races are run to benefit a cause, like Komen's Race for the Cure, which benefits the fight against women's cancers. Running for a cause is a great reason to run! Look in the Resources section for a list of organizations that have national fund-raising races.

As you know by now, I'm training for my fourth marathon. And to be completely honest, I signed up for it not necessarily because I wanted to run the painful race again. In fact, I'm looking forward to the day it's over. But, after moving across the country and adjusting to a new lifestyle and schedule out here in California, I was having a hard time running regularly. I hadn't gotten into a

> *Running's a priority for me, because the rest of my day's better if I run. I just make it a priority. Instead of getting a little more sleep, I run.*
>
> Laura, 36

routine and knew that I needed to do something to jump-start my running again. Well, signing up for a four-and-a-half-hour run did it. I printed out a training schedule and entered into my calendar the days I was to run and what the distance was. Now, every morning when I get to work and turn on my computer, I get this little reminder in the upper right-hand corner, prodding me to run that day's distance. And I know that the marathon is going to be pretty darn difficult if I don't get my runs in. Enough said. I'm running. After the marathon, it will be time to set my sights on some new running goals. And then I'll keep on running. (See chapter Ten for more information on running road races.)

Run with a Dog

Ari B. Reber is my puppy. Well, he's a 12½-year-old collie/shepherd mix, so I guess technically speaking he's not a puppy anymore. I adopted him when I was a sophomore in college, picking him from a whole litter of puppies at a farm in central Pennsylvania. He was about four years old when I moved to New York City, admittedly not the best place to raise a family, let alone a 60-pound dog. That's when Ari started running with me. I loved the companionship of having him along. I loved the pride I felt when people passing by on their in-line skates would comment or smile at my dog's wonderfulness. I loved the security I felt by having him by my side. And I loved the fact that I felt like I was being a good mom (I have no children, so being my dog's primary caregiver is as close as I've come to motherhood thus far). It was a win-win situation. Sure,

The best thing about running with Gunther is that I feel like we're doing the all-American thing. Like we should be on a postcard or something. Plus, I'm doing something great for him and me at the same time.
Amy, 30

Ari would occasionally catch a whiff of an amazingly wonderful scent and feel the need to drag me with all his might in a direction other than the one all of my momentum was moving in, and we would conduct our own personal game of tug-of-war, which I *usually* won. But for the most part, his companionship during my runs was a great thing.

Ari stopped running with me about five years ago. One afternoon we were doing the loop around the reservoir, and when we finished and started to walk home, I noticed Ari was limping slightly. I took him to the vet and she told me it was probably time to end Ari's running career, as he was getting old and was starting to suffer from arthritis. She said that Ari would rather keel over dead than not keep up with me, and if I kept bringing him along for runs, he might just do that. But it was good while it lasted.

I know there are lots of readers out there who don't have a dog. So I say, borrow one! Back when Ari was still running, I actually lent him to a friend for runs. My friend missed his own dog, who was with his parents, and he liked the bonding time with Ari. And Ari, well, he just wanted to run.

Mind Games and Rituals

Sometimes I make myself focus on my breathing and try to block out other things. I also set lots of small goals, like to make it to the tree up ahead. And then once I pass it, I do it all over again.
Sarah, 28

While many of the motivational suggestions in this chapter have to do with keeping you going from one run to the next, here we deal more with how to keep going once you start a run. How to get through a run when you're not in the mood is an important skill to have. If we changed into our running clothes, headed out the door, and one mile into a five-mile run decided we weren't in the mood and turned around, then obviously something isn't working right. Not that I haven't done exactly that. I have, and on more than one occasion. But if that behavior becomes the norm, then making running a permanent part of our lives is going to be a difficult proposal.

One way I keep myself going is to play mind games when I run. The type of game varies from run to run. Perhaps the one I play most often, as does my husband (and Tip, too, I recently discovered), is a math game highlighting the wonders of fractions. I talked about this a bit in the section on running on tracks, but really it applies to any run. Math is a great thing to focus on, because it's a complete and utter distraction from the task at hand.

Here's an example. When Derin and I were running a half-marathon in Fresno a few months ago (his first), I was wearing my watch, which only stored up to eight splits, or laps. That wasn't going to cut it if I wanted to keep track of our mile splits, because there would be thirteen. Now, in keeping with my anal-retentive and overly organized personality, I'm a very technical runner. Meaning, I have to know exactly (down to the second) what pace I'm running when I'm doing a race or long-distance run. So, after we finished the first mile of this run, I checked my watch. It read 10:35. I wanted to run a ten-and-a-half-minute mile for the next mile, so I did the math in my head, and figured out that by the next mile my watch should read 21:05. And depending on how close I was to hitting that mark, I would adjust my pace accordingly. Of course, I'd then spend some time figuring out exactly how much of the race I

I always give myself an out. I can turn around and go home after five minutes if it still feels terrible. That typically doesn't happen.
Beth, 35

had completed. At the first mile I would be 1/13 of the way done. Then I'd determine what my projected finishing time was if I kept up this pace. And so on. That's a good one to two minutes per mile that I'm not consciously aware of because I'm caught up with doing math in my head.

Not all mind games have to be this intense, nor do they have to involve math. Sometimes I simply sing songs in my head. During one New York City Marathon, which I ran alone, I sang the entire Indigo Girls album *Indians, Nomads and Saints* in my head. Kind of maddening, but I figured that the album was nearly an hour long, and it would get me through an hour of the marathon.

I define rituals as the little things we all do as a way of being ourselves. Think about things you do every day, like brush your teeth, or dry your hair or feed the dog. We all have little things we do that make those moments uniquely ours. Running rituals work the same way. My husband actually started one ritual that I eventually joined him in because I loved it. Remember that steep hill in Central Park called Cat Hill? Well, every time we would run up that hill, Derin would yell out, "Thank you, cat!" as if he were thanking the cat goddess of the hill for giving him the strength to make it to the top. I soon realized that I'd better start thanking the cat, too, lest the cat think me ungrateful and start making the hill unbearably difficult to conquer. Rituals can be as simple as which side of the road or path you want to run

on when with a partner. Or always sprinting when you reach a certain spot. Or maybe stopping for water at a scenic water fountain and stretching. Whatever you can do to own the run and make it special to you will ultimately help you get through the run, from start to finish.

Be Flexible (and Forgiving)

Above all, be flexible with yourself and your running program. Not every run will be wonderful, and there will be days when you don't want to run at all. That's okay! Allow yourself days off. And allow yourself runs that feel terrible. And allow yourself the room to be flexible. Sometimes the best-laid plans can fall through. What you want to avoid is reaching a point where running feels like a chore and you begin to dread your workouts. If your goal is to make running a permanent part of your life, accept that there will be good days and there will be bad days. Days off here and there, even a few weeks if you're starting to feel burned out, can be a healthy part of your running program.

I find that I go through phases where I'm more excited or less excited about running. And if I'm in a phase where I'm less excited, then I mix it up with something else.
Christie, 29

9

Safety First:

Running Safely, Running Injury-Free

As you know by now, I believe that running is an incredibly empowering thing for women to do. So when I hear about a woman runner being assaulted, I am deeply affected. I get sad and angry. One night about a mile into a run in Central Park, I stumbled upon a crime scene, flooded with cops, park rangers and detectives, all looking for evidence relating to the murder of a woman jogger earlier that morning. The next thing I knew, I was brushing back tears. I was so caught off guard that I had to stop running and catch my breath. All I kept thinking was how dare someone attack a woman who was out here running, out here doing something to make herself stronger. Running is good for the soul. For anyone to give women a reason to be afraid to run is a horrible crime in itself.

That next day, I called up the New York Road Runners Club and asked them if there was anything they were doing, or if there was anything I could do to prevent something like this from happening again. The Club suggested I stop by and pick up one of their safety brochures, which I did. But, I wanted to do more. I wanted to start some sort of kick-ass women's organization that would patrol the park and find the person(s) who did this crime. To this day, the murder has gone unsolved. And my early evening runs in the park were never the same. This is probably a good thing, since it's not a good idea to become too comfortable in our surroundings when running no matter where we are. It's a sad state of reality, but that's the way it is. But that doesn't mean we have to be sitting ducks for potential harm. In fact, the things I learned through the Road Runners Club's safety guidelines brochure are tips that have allowed me to continue running alone, and enjoy my runs to the fullest. The safety recommendations below come from the RRCA guidelines for women runners.

Safety Tips for Women Runners

- Don't wear headsets

- Carry a quarter

- Run with a partner

- Leave word when and where you're running

- Run in familiar areas

- Run in populated areas

- Carry ID

- Don't wear jewelry

- Ignore verbal harassment

- Run against traffic

- Wear reflective material

- Practice memorizing license plates and characteristics of strangers

- Carry a noisemaker or pepper spray

- Use your intuition

Don't Wear Headsets

Many women run with headphones, plugged into tapes or CDs, or in my case, the radio. Music can be a great tool to make a workout go faster or keep you motivated while you run. I ran with a radio for years when I ran outdoors, and listened to music at my gym in the basement of UNICEF, where I worked. But the first year I decided to run outdoors year round, I knew I needed to make a change. As someone who always used to run after work during the week, daylight savings time pretty much guaranteed that any run in the winter would be after dark. And Central Park at night can become an eerie ghost town of sorts. So, I decided to stop running with headphones over the winter. The reasons are pretty obvious. When listening to music I was making myself really vulnerable. I wouldn't be able to hear someone approaching from behind me, or be aware of possible trouble up ahead. Part of the whole idea of running with music

I was assaulted when I was jogging about four years ago. I was on a bike path and wearing my Walkman, and a guy came up behind me because I didn't hear him. Now I never run with a Walkman.
Sarah, 28

is that you can kind of "zone out" while you run. But zoning out when running alone at night isn't such a good idea.

This doesn't mean that running during the daylight with your headphones at full blast is a great idea either. In fact, the RRCA recommends that women never run outdoors with headphones—there are just too many risks. Ideally, you should always be able to hear some outside noise. In Central Park, bikers would come flying around corners and yell "on your right!" at joggers who were off in their own world. And I've seen runners hit from behind by bikers because they didn't yield to their warnings.

Carry a Quarter

It's always a great idea to carry a quarter with you in case you find yourself needing to make a call at a payphone. That quarter is your connection to the outside world when you run. Don't leave home without it. Also, keep your eyes open for emergency phones. A lot of city parks have phones placed throughout the park that require no change and instantly connect the caller with the police, kind of like the President's special red phone. On your next run, take note of any emergency or payphones along your route. Most running shorts or tights have a little pocket on the inside under the waistband that's the perfect size for a quarter. And as cell phones get smaller and lighter, you could also consider running with one in your pocket or fanny pack.

Run with a Partner

There are many benefits to running with a partner, and safety is a big one. Beyond Frank's and my respective breakups as an impetus to our running together, the fact that we were able to run later at night than I might have alone was a great thing. People out to do others harm invariably go for the easy target. Running with a partner definitely decreases your chances of being attacked.

Leave Word When and Where You're Running

I believe in being a safe runner, so I make sure that I leave behind a note for my boyfriend or roommate about where I'm running and the estimated time it will take me, just so people know where I am.
Emily, 29

This is a really important consideration, especially if you're running alone. When I go for runs by myself, and Derin isn't home from work yet, I always leave a note for him with the time I left for my run, my planned route and the time I think I'll be back. Simple enough, and it makes me feel better about running alone. Even if you don't live with a roommate, it's a good idea to leave this information on a Post-it by your telephone or some other visible place in your home.

Run in Familiar Areas

Sometimes going out on a run with no real plan as to where your feet may take you can breathe new life into a run. But even if this is your plan, make sure not to stray into new neighborhoods that you haven't driven through first or aren't familiar with. There are too many unknowns, including unleashed dogs and the potential is always there to find yourself in a dodgy neighborhood.

Sometimes you can't always be familiar with the neighborhoods you're running in, particularly if you go for a run when you're traveling. So make sure that someone knows your route, be it a friend or a clerk at the hotel front desk.

I don't run when it's dark out. I used to, and I don't do it anymore. And I make sure to run on the main road if it's early in the morning.
Laura, 36

Run in Populated Areas

There is a traverse in Central Park at 102nd Street called, appropriately enough, the 102nd Street Traverse. As part of my four-mile loop, I used to cut across this traverse, which took me from the east to the west side of the park, and thankfully allowed me to skip a brutal downhill and steep uphill at the north end of the park. The traverse itself has some history—it was the site of the infamous brutal attack of the Central Park Jogger in 1989—where a young woman was gang-raped and beaten by a group of youths on a "wilding spree." Nine years later, it was the locale for the murder mentioned at the beginning of this chapter. Since that latter murder, the NYPD stationed a police vehicle halfway between the east and west side entrances. The half-mile road was closed to traffic, and unlike the outside loop around the park, it could be very quiet and spooky. Several times while running alone after dark I would cross this traverse, sprinting until I saw the police vehicle's lights on and heard the motor running. Then I sprinted again to the exit on the west side once I was out of plain view of the police car. Scary. And not smart. I stopped doing this after one night when I did my first half sprint only to

I generally feel okay running alone in the park, because I go in the morning when there are a lot of people out.
Emily, 30

find that the police vehicle was nowhere to be found. So I kept on sprinting. And I was exhausted by the time I got to the other side. That was the last time I ran the traverse alone at night. It just wasn't worth the anxiety or the risk.

Carry ID

I usually carry three pieces of ID with me: my license, my credit card and my medical insurance card.
Colleen, 26

Most of us don't want to run around with our driver's license shoved in our shoe or running bra. But the RRCA's advice is to write your personal information in permanent ink on the inside sole of your running shoe. They recommend you include your name, telephone number, and blood type. And if you have any other pertinent medical information, you should include that, too.

Don't Wear Jewelry

When you snorkel where there are barracudas, you're supposed to take off all of your jewelry before you get in the water. Apparently barracudas are attracted to shiny movements in the water, and they've been known to bite ears and fingers because they were drawn to someone's earring or ring. The same logic applies to running. Wearing jewelry when you run makes yourself a more likely target for someone wanting to do you harm. When I run alone, I do sometimes run with my wedding ring, but I often turn my sapphire stone inward toward my palm if I'm feeling uncomfortable. Since I usually run with my husband or my neighbor, I usually feel comfortable keeping it on, but again, use your instincts.

Ignore Verbal Harrassment

Oh boy, do I have a hard time with this one. Verbal harassment is one of my huge pet peeves. If I were a public advocate, I'd make verbal harassment a seriously punishable crime. By verbal harassment I'm talking about men who feel the need to make comments to women—on our appearance, our breasts, our smile. In fact, there have been many times when I've told men verbally harassing me on the sidewalks of New York exactly what they could do with themselves. I know this is not a good idea, and it's an even worse idea when running. And I've done my best to change my approach. As a runner, you'll inevitably find yourself the victim of some sort of verbal harassment, whether it's some person telling you "faster, faster" as you run past him (of course, he's out of shape, walking slowly and shoving his fifth hotdog of the day in his mouth), or being whistled at and admired for your runner's legs, butt or your bouncing chest. Just let it go.

If people are harassing me, I assume the best. I just assume that they're saying something positive. Or I just ignore it and keep going.
Bridget, 32

Run Against Traffic

This is something I learned a long time ago. I think it must have been my high school cross-country coach, Whitney Seltzer, who first explained the importance of running facing traffic before sending us out for our longer runs. The upside of running against traffic is that you can see people coming toward you and visa versa. Unless you're running on a sidewalk or on a running path that prohibits cars, running against traffic is one of the golden rules of running. This is especially impor-

I have three or four different routes that I run. I tell my husband which one I'm on, so he knows which direction I go and how long it will take me.
Karen, 39

tant if you're running at night. Drivers might not be expecting to share the road with you.

Wear Reflective Material

This is another important consideration for any night runners. Most running shoes these days come with some sort of reflective material on them. You might not notice how bright this is until you're driving along and your headlights shine on a pair of runners' shoes or a vest. They'll light up like a Christmas tree. And it's not just shoes that contain reflective material. Many runners' tights have reflective strips along the back, and jackets also tend to have strips of reflective material. If you really want to get fancy, you can wear a runner's vest that looks like a safety patrol vest . . . bright colors with thick reflective material all around. Regardless of what the outfit, wearing reflective gear is an easy way to keep yourself out of harm's way when running after dark.

Practice Memorizing License Plates or Characteristics of Strangers

I pay attention to strangers when I'm running. I adopt the same sort of awareness around me as when I'm walking. And I don't let anyone run behind me. I'm very aware of my surroundings. AnneMarie, 32

This may seem like an odd recommendation, but it works. We used to tease my friend in college about his many neuroses, one of which was memorizing license plates. That was just something he did, particularly on cars that looked "suspicious" to him for whatever reason. My roommate and I thought this was really funny at the time. Now, of course, I have my own weird neuroses, one of which involves looking out for low-flying airplanes and noting the time and place where I saw them. Don't ask. But the point is, observation skills can be honed, and memorizing license plates or characteristics of strangers can be a valuable skill in case of any incidents with runners. In the Upper East Side of Manhattan, a rapist has been on the loose since 1996 despite the fact that his mug shot is plastered all over every bodega and subway station in the neighborhood. It seems like people today are so caught up in their own lives, they're too busy to notice things going on around them. But when running, stay alert and keep your eyes out for anything out of the ordinary. Try to remember as much detail as possible. It could prove valuable down the road.

Carry a Noisemaker or Pepper Spray

This is something that the RRCA recommends, but with the caveat that you should be trained in the use of pepper spray before taking it out with you, as it's pretty potent stuff. There are a lot of small noisemakers out there that make a loud, harsh, obnoxious sound when set off, and one that would probably cause a potential attacker to reconsider his plan. I personally don't carry a noisemaker or pepper spray, although I have run with Mace before.

I have to take precautions because I run first thing in the morning. I wear a reflective vest, I have pepper spray that I clip onto my belt and I'm also very careful about my route.
Paulette, 50

Use Your Intuition

This is probably the most important thing for us all to remember. Listen to that little voice inside of you. If something about a situation just doesn't feel right, then chances are, it's not. There are so many occasions when we do things out of fear of embarrassment or because we want to prove how tough we are. Well, there's no such thing as embarrassment when our safety is at stake. If I'm running alone at night and I hear some-one running up behind me, I jerk my head around to make sure it's another runner. And if it's a male runner, oftentimes I'll cross the street, or move way to the side so he can pass me. Sometimes I feel a little paranoid doing this, but I'd rather be perceived as paranoid than be assaulted.

During my last summer in New York, I found myself in a sit-uation where I was forced to use my intuition, and it didn't let me down. I had just finished a run in Central Park on a sunny Sunday afternoon, and as I crossed the street to exit the park I noticed that a biker I had seen earlier on my run had stopped, and was pushing his bike across the street in my direction. I'm not sure what caused me to pay attention to this man, but something about the situation heightened my senses. As I made my way toward my apartment, I heard the sound of bike wheels behind me, so I started to jog. I heard the biker get on his bike and continue following me at about the same distance. Over the next few blocks, I crossed streets diagonally, and made some pretty last-minute turns, and still the biker fol-lowed me at every turn. I was nearing my apartment and didn't know exactly what to do, so I turned into a deli to call my hus-band. As I entered the store, I saw the biker pull his bike along-side the building next door and dismount. I made a beeline to the back of the store, and called my husband from the store phone. I waited in the back and saw the biker enter the store, obviously looking for me as he moved around the side of a display shelf. I stepped to the other side just as Derin walked in the door, grabbed my hand, and we snuck out before the guy had a chance to see us leave. We walked for blocks and blocks in the opposite direction of our apartment, making sure that we lost him. I was really shaken by the whole thing. But because I followed my instincts and made some good decisions, I got through the situation relatively unscathed. So, listen to that little voice inside of you. It's often right.

Safety and the Elements

Depending on the weather and the running conditions you encounter on any given day, you should be aware of some of the ways the elements can adversely affect our bodies. Usually these are things that need to be considered when dealing with extreme circumstances, such as extreme heat or cold, or running faster than usual. But with the right awareness and preparation, you can fend off any of these potential problems before they become serious.

Warm Weather Running

During a five-mile race in Central Park, I rounded the corner near the finish line to see a bunch of race officials attending to a man lying along the side of the road against the embankment. It looked like he was passed out cold. They were pouring water on his head and generally looking pretty alarmed. They were. The man was suffering from heat exhaustion, which means that his

I'm really fair-skinned, so sunburn is something I have to be really careful about. I have to apply sunscreen diligently and always carry some with me. Sarah, 28

body's cooling system had become overheated and his internal body temperature had become dangerously high.

Heatstroke and heat exhaustion can happen anytime, and not just to runners. They are usually the result of intense exertion in really hot conditions—essentially the body just overheats. Heat exhaustion is the more common and less serious of the two ailments. Usually a person suffering from heat exhaustion is overcome by weakness and dizziness, and even disorientation. In many cases it is a result of the body sweating out so much fluid that the person can't replenish it fast enough, and the body overheats. I have come close to suffering from heat exhaustion at times. During several races in extremely hot conditions, I found myself getting dizzy while running. Sometimes I would get a chill, and then realize that I'm not sweating. Bad sign. This is when I slow down and get some water. Anytime I'm running in ninety-degree temperatures and there's no sweat pouring from my body, I know something is wrong.

Heatstroke is more serious, and can be lethal if not treated immediately. A person suffering from heatstroke will generally start breathing rapidly, and their heart rate will skyrocket. Their body temperature could shoot as high as 106 degrees Fahrenheit, and they could become unconscious. If not treated immediately to lower the body temperature, the person could suffer from permanent brain damage or even die.

Both heat exhaustion and heatstroke are extreme conditions, and can be avoided by listening to your body and being aware of the onset of any of these symptoms: dizziness, muscle cramps, nausea, lack of sweating in high temperatures or profuse sweating, thirst and light-headedness.

📖 **Heat Exhaustion** is the overheating of the body from loss of water, and is accompanied by headache, dizziness and nausea.

📖 **Heatstroke** is more severe and is a result of the body's internal temperature regulator malfunctioning, and symptoms can include disorientation, rapid heart rate and quick breathing.

Dehydration is similar in some ways to heat exhaustion in that it's directly caused by the body not having enough fluids. Many of us go day-to-day, even when we're not exercising, in a state of dehydration, because we simply don't drink as much water as we should. They say that if you're thirsty, you're already dehydrated. The point is, you can never drink too much water. If you're running the next morning, be sure to drink an ample amount of water the night before. If you're running a race, be sure to drink several cups of water before you even begin, and drink more along the way at water stops. And, of course, when you finish any run, drink drink drink.

When I'm running in hot weather, I always have water with me and make sure I'm hydrated. I usually pour water on my body and my head if I'm really hot. Christie, 29

If you don't have enough fluids in your body, you can become physically dehydrated, which can involve being dizzy and confused, accompanied by a low blood pressure. Dehydration is nothing to mess around with, and especially when running in hot weather, you can

TIPS FOR RUNNING IN EXTREME HEAT AND HUMIDITY

- Stay properly hydrated
- Don't overexert yourself
- Wear loose, cool, light-colored clothing
- Listen to your body
- Do less intense workouts

become dehydrated very quickly and without warning, putting you at risk for heat exhaustion or heatstroke. If you're suffering from dehydration, in all but the mildest of cases, you should go to the hospital and get some intravenous fluids. It's the quickest, most direct way to replenish your body.

Cold Weather Running

The biggest concern when running in extremely cold weather is frostbite. Anything that is exposed to the harsh, cold winter air is at risk, and since frostbite will leave you feeling numb, you may not even realize that you're in danger. Take proper care to cover your hands, head, ears and as much of your face as possible when running in extremely cold conditions. It is especially important to cover up during sleet, snow or when the windchill drops the temperature below the freezing mark. Play it safe and if the weather is questionably cold, bring the hats and gloves. You can take them off and stick them in your pocket if you become overheated.

> Running in the rain can be great, but if there's lightning in the area, take your run inside.

Cold weather can bring other obstacles, particularly snow and ice. If you're a year round outdoor runner, be especially careful when running on these surfaces, as a slick ice patch can be extremely dangerous to a runner. When running you have all of your body's momentum moving forward, which makes it harder to get control if you're slipping on some ice. If you do manage to catch yourself you could strain a muscle, or worse. If you have to run in the snow or ice, wear a trail shoe with a substantial tread.

One time I slipped on the ice in the winter and tore a muscle in the inside of my thigh. So I had to bite the bullet and do upper body exercises for a while and get through it the best I could.
Janet, 51

Injuries, Aches And Pains

While running isn't exactly a dangerous sport, there are some ailments that can affect runners more so than people participating in other sports. Here is a breakdown of some of the more common conditions that affect runners. This isn't a complete list of every possible muscle or bone injury that you may encounter as a result of running or any other physical exercise. For more details on specific injuries, I recommend getting a copy of *Runner's World's Sports Medicine Guide,* or visiting their website at *www.runnersworld.com.*

Running Feet—Blisters and More

The day that I'm writing this, I just pulled off a huge hunk of skin from my little pinky toe, the leftover reminder of a blister as deep as the Grand Canyon. Kind of gross I know, but blisters are a part of running long distances for many runners. You might not think of blisters as being especially problematic or even painful for that matter, but I've had some whoppers in my day, including the one I bid *sayonara* to this morning. Both blisters and calluses are common plagues of the runner's foot.

The good news is, there are precautions you can take to avoid getting blisters and calluses in the first place. The wonders of Vaseline come into play here—before any long run, rub a small amount of Vaseline between and around your toes, your heel and any other blister-prone areas. There are also products out there made specifically to prevent blisters that you can use instead of

I trained last year for a half-marathon and tore the Plantaris in my foot. I had to scale back for a while. Now I run with orthotics, but it hasn't slowed me down.
Karen, 39

Vaseline, such as Runner's Lube, Sportslick or BodyGlide. And since blisters and calluses are caused by friction, the fit of your shoe or the type of sock you're running in can make a difference as well. Shoes that are too big or small can work against you—you don't want to be sliding around, but you don't want to have to squeeze your foot in either. Wearing socks that are designed to keep your foot dry and breathe out the sweat that will inevitably occur down there is another great way to prevent blisters and calluses. CoolMax socks are known for their ability to keep feet nice and dry. It will make a big difference.

> I'm a Pisces, so I generally have foot ailments. I used to get huge calluses from running, but after I learned more about how I ran and changed my shoes to ones that were more padded up front, they went away.
> AnneMarie, 32

But despite all of this good planning, I still sometimes discover a huge bubble of a blister on the bottom of a toe after a run, and you might, too. I prefer to pop the blister with a pin—after heating the end to sterilize it. Popping blisters tends to relieve the immediate discomfort and allow you to go on with your day. But lately I've been using blister guards from Band-Aid. These little pads help the blistered area to heal while protecting it from further problems.

Black toenails are another common foot ailment. Ah. Black toenails. That's an attractive thought, isn't it? Black toenails don't affect everyone, but the longer your runs, the better your chance of developing these. I've had black toenails three times in my life—once after each marathon. The black is actually dried blood underneath the nail, and it's usually a result of continual pressure on the toe because of shoes that fit poorly, or rubbing during a really long run. In my case, the black toenail also develops a blister underneath it, which I drain with a sterilized needle. Eventually, the toenail falls off. This sounds painful, but it's actually not at all. And the weird thing is that there's always a brand-new toenail growing underneath. The body is an amazing thing.

Another foot problem I'm currently suffering from is athlete's foot, again, a pretty common condition among runners. It's a fungus (yuck) on the bottom of your feet that causes redness and irritation and can be quite uncomfortable. Like most ailments, prevention is the best medicine, and running in cotton, breathable socks is a good way to stave off this infection. If you get athlete's foot, you can buy topical solution at any drugstore to cure it.

Plantar Fasciitis

More serious than these other foot ailments is plantar fasciitis, which is when a fibrous band along the bottom of the foot stretches and tears, and your foot feels almost as though the bone is bruised. The causes for plantar fasciitis are varied—anything from a severe overpronation to running in shoes that have lost their spring. I developed plantar fasciitis years ago because I was running in a motion-control shoe when I didn't need to. The shoe held my foot so rigidly that the fiber band was being constantly tugged and stretched. Once I figured out what was going on, I switched to a less restrictive pair of running shoes, and after a short break from running, the symptoms went away. If you are faced with this ailment, some time off, combined with icing the area to reduce inflammation, should take care of the problem. You could also look into getting a different running shoe. If the problem persists, you may want to visit a podiatrist, who can fit you for insoles for your running shoes, which should address this problem.

When I first started running, I used to get black toenails, but I think it was the sneakers. Since I switched shoes, it hasn't happened. Emily, 30

Iliotibial Band Syndrome (ITBS)

My ITBS is a real bummer, because it stopped me from running the marathon this year. But on the other hand, after periods where I haven't been able to run at all, I'm just happy that I can get back out there.
Christie, 29

Iliotibial Band Syndrome, or ITBS as it's known among us sufferers, is something I know all too much about. I first developed this common runner's problem in 1996 after running my first marathon. I was running a 10k in the park about a month later, and had to pull out of the race because of excruciating pain in my outer knee area. I did what most people in my situation would do. I panicked, thinking that I had seriously damaged my knee and went off to see an orthopedist. He told me I didn't have any cartilage damage to my knee, and suggested I take a break from running for a while. I did. But when I started up again, I still had that same pain in my knee, and a similar burning discomfort in my outer hip socket. A woman I worked with recommended I go see her chiropractor, and he diagnosed my ITBS.

The last long training run I did I had problems with my hip, and what got me through it was my running buddy and ibuprofen.
Karen, 36

The iliotibial band is a band of fiber that connects the outside of the knee socket to the outside of the hip socket. The syndrome is caused when that fiber band tightens up. When I went to see the chiropractor, even the slightest amount of pressure along any point of my outer thigh was extremely sensitive. I didn't even know it hurt because I hadn't touched it before then. I went through a whole process of therapy—biweekly electrotherapy on my knee, ultrasound on my hip, massages, stretches, ice and worst of all, no running. I did this for about a month and a half. And it didn't get any better. It felt great while I was having these treatments done, but my knee still hurt a lot when walking down stairs, and I couldn't lie on my side in bed, let alone run.

So, I started to do some research. I found out that ITBS is really common among runners, and is commonly misdiagnosed as runner's knee. No one is sure what exactly causes it (my chiropractor thought it was because my legs were uneven, and had me wear a lift in one of my shoes for a while. This didn't help and I haven't worn one since). Some of the other potential causes include scaling up miles too quickly, wearing inappropriate workout shoes, being inflexible and running downhill. Regardless of the cause, the symptoms are usually the same: a dull, aching pain in the outer hip socket/butt area, and then more severe, sharp pain in the outer knee socket area. These areas, along with the IT band itself, are sensitive to the touch.

The solution that I've found works best for this syndrome is simple—stretching. Since ITBS is caused by a tightening of the iliotibial band, keeping it loose and flexible is the key. ITBS stretches (described in detail in Chapter four) should be done before and after running, and even on days that you don't run at all. If you're still experiencing problems after concentrating on stretching the band, you may need to take some time off from running, or run shorter distances for a while until the pain starts to go away. Icing the area that hurts is also an option. If it continues to be severe you may need to visit a doctor to talk about possible remedies. Five years after I first contracted ITBS, it's still a part of my life. I can't run without stretching my IT band, and I still have problems sleeping directly on my hip for too long. But I'm able to run pain free, and that's the important thing.

Charley Horse

If you've ever gotten a charley horse (a fancy name for a leg cramp), you know how painful these muscle spasms can be. The first time I experienced this was back when I was in the ninth grade or so. I woke up in the middle of the night screaming in pain and clutching my calf. My calf muscle had balled itself up into a little knot high in my lower leg, and the pain was excruciating. My dad ran over to my room and helped to massage out the cramp, but in the morning I could barely walk on it. It remained sore for about two days.

The best thing to do about charley horses is to prevent them. For me, they usually happen after intense workouts when my muscles are tight to begin with. If I go to bed without doing some extra stretching, I may inadvertently cause the cramp while I'm sleeping by turning or straightening out my leg too quickly. If you're prone to tight muscles, make sure to spend some time massaging them, or even use a sports cream like BenGay to help keep the muscle warm and loose.

Shinsplints

Many people have experienced shinsplints at some point in their life—it's another one of those ailments that affects lots of people, not just runners. Shinsplints are a painful condition along the inside, outside or front of the shinbone. If you have shinsplints, you'll feel a burning sensation at some point along the shinbone, depending on where it's affecting you. I used to get shinsplints regularly when I ran track, and would have to tape up my legs to get through a meet.

In many cases, shinsplints are caused by running on

> **R.I.C.E. is a traditional remedy for an inflammation or swelling caused by running. It stands for Rest, Ice, Compression and Elevation.**

extremely hard surfaces, like cement or tarmac. You can also get them by running up or down steep hills, which places a big strain on this part of the leg, or by running in shoes that aren't cushioned enough. The best way to deal with shinsplints is to prevent them, and the best way to do this is to run on softer surfaces, like grass or dirt or cinder, and run on flat surfaces with only mild inclinations. Once you've got shinsplints, you'll be uncomfortable even walking. If you do find yourself with shinsplints, try icing them—this keeps the inflammation down, which is causing the pain. Take Dixie cups and fill them with water and stick them in the freezer. After they're frozen, tear off the top half of the cup and you now have an instant ice massager. Ice your shins a couple of times a day if the pain is severe and take a break from running for a few days, or longer if the pain persists. When you do start up again, make sure that you run on soft surfaces for a while.

Sore Nipples and Chafing

Ah, here is another opportunity to experience the wonders of Vaseline. Just as it works in preventing blisters and calluses, Vaseline can help prevent uncomfortable rubbing in other areas as well. I only learned about runner's nipple about four years ago. I noticed that sometimes after taking off my running bra after a long run, my nipples would be extremely sen-

sitive, and very painful to the touch. I usually noticed this
more when I was cold and had worn a lot of layers. I assumed
it was the result of my nipples being cold and erect for so
long. Or something like that. I now know about runner's nipple, which is a common condition among women *and* men. It
is caused by the friction of the nipple against a running bra or
T-shirt, which causes chafing and hence, pain. I have seen
men running with two bloodstains on their shirts where their
nipples are and I want to pass them a jar of Vaseline right then
and there. You may not find this is a problem in shorter runs,
but when I'm running over six miles I always put Vaseline on
my nipples to prevent this painful condition.

Other areas prone to chafing are the armpit and the inside
leg area. Vaseline works just as well here. Be aware though, if
you use Vaseline in your armpit in combination with deodorant, you'll eventually have a white foamy-looking substance
around the armpit area—something about the mixing of
deodorant, Vaseline and sweat. But hey, it's the price you pay
for a chafe-free run.

Runner's Knee

When I tell people that I'm a runner, people often say they've
got bad knees, so they're afraid to run. Knees seem to be of
major concern among runners and nonrunners alike. So what
is runner's knee? The technical name for it is Chondromalacia
Patellae, and it is the eroding of the kneecap and cartilage
around it. If you experience significant pain in and around the

kneecap area, along with some swelling, you may want to talk to a doctor and get a diagnosis.

The best way to deal with any injury is to prevent it. Making sure you're running in properly cushioned running shoes can go a long way toward preventing runner's knee. Another recommendation is to keep your quadriceps muscles strong by doing leg lifts or other such weight training, to help make your running gait more efficient and reduce the risk of unnecessary strain on the knee.

I've had several knee surgeries, but what's interesting is that I don't notice any correlation between running and pain in my knee. Sometimes I've found when my knee's been bothering me and I go running, it actually feels better.
Bridget, 32

Side Stitches

Side stitches are painful cramps that can occur anywhere in the mid-section, generally near your diaphragm. The absolute cause of side stitches isn't known, nor is there foolproof information regarding prevention and remedy. Eating or drinking immediately before running, and improper breathing while exercising have both been linked to this ailment.

My high school track coach taught me a technique of applying firm pressure directly on the cramp and inhaling deeply, while either continuing to run slowly or stopping to walk. This sometimes works. And as I said earlier, inhaling through the nose and exhaling out the mouth as a normal breathing pattern while running has also decreased the number of side stitches I get in general. The *Runner's World's Sports Medicine Guide* recommends taking in a deep breath, holding it and then puckering your lips to force the air out.

If the stitch is dull, you might be able to run through it, and it will eventually go away. But sharp side stitches can be crippling—when they're really severe I have to stop and walk. I'll reach a point where even the slightest movement or shift in my upper body will be painful, and this makes running nearly impossible.

The Key to Injury Is Prevention

As always, prevention is the best remedy for any injury or ailment. And listen to your body. If you're experiencing pain, try to qualify it. Is it sharp or dull? Is it soreness or more? Are you alarmed? Then think about whether you've changed anything in your running pattern that might have caused the symptoms you're feeling, such as new running shoes or running longer or faster than usual. If something feels off for you, oftentimes it's the direct result of some change you've made in your routine. Use your common sense. If the pain continues and you're alarmed, visit a doctor and get a diagnosis.

Most important, take care of your body! Stretch and warm up your muscles before any run, and engage in other activities like weight training to keep your whole body fine-tuned. The better overall shape you're in and the more well-rounded your fitness, the less likely you'll find yourself on the injured roster.

10.

On Your Mark:

Are Road Races for You?

Since the age of five, I've been involved in sports. First gymnastics, and then track-and-field in middle school. You could say that competition is part of my life. So, when I quit the track team at Penn State after a year of struggling (and I mean *struggling*) as a walk-on, the hardest part for me to swallow was believing that my racing days were over. No more nervous stomach in anticipation of the gun going off, no more psyching myself up with music (the sound track to *Chariots of Fire* was my favorite) and no more competition. It wasn't until about six years later that I signed up for a local 5K (3.1 miles) race.

When I showed up the morning of the race, I couldn't believe how many people were there. Literally thousands of men and women, and some kids, had gotten up at seven A.M. just to run a race! And these weren't necessarily competitive runners, or runners who had been athletes their whole lives. The field of runners ran the gamut, from walkers to casual joggers to the leaders of the pack. The whole experience was awesome. I ran right in the middle of the pack, talking with other runners, groaning with them on the hills and having just enough energy left at the finish to sprint the last hundred or so yards. That was it for me. I was hooked. In the big monster of a city that is New York, I had found a community. Eight years later, I still run about a dozen road races a year.

What to Expect When You're Racing

Tell someone you're running a race and you'll get all different kinds of reactions. Some shrink away in horror at the thought, others are just plain old baffled, as if pondering the question, "Why on earth would anyone willingly submit themselves to such torture?" I think it's the word *race* itself that turns off so many people, maybe even yourself. So maybe it's best to think about races in other terms.

Supported Group Runs

Before I go into all the wonderful, positive things about racing, I thought maybe it would be worth talking about races in general to help dispel the fears of the unknown. Road races are essentially *supported group runs*. They are always sponsored by an organization (or many different ones), and these sponsors are responsible for providing all of the "support." At any road race you'll find things to make your run easier, like water stations along the route. The number of water stations depends on the length of the run. Usually, these will be placed every two miles or so, and there will be lots of helpful volunteers standing next to the tables holding cups for you to grab as you run by. They're also there to sweep up all the discarded cups along the route.

Another form of support is that the course will be a truly measured route. Most of the runs I have around my neighborhood are guesstimated distances. Unless I'm running around a track, I don't ever know for sure the exact distance I'm running or my exact running pace. But along a measured route, you can be assured that the total distance of the race, as well as each mile from start to finish, will be marked. And usually, the race sponsors will even have people standing at each mile marker to yell out your time as you pass by, or they'll have large digital timers in place.

And then there are the portable toilets. Granted, the nervous stomachs and bladders many runners experience before a race make portable bathrooms more important than during a normal solo run, but they're still good to have around. Just be aware that a lot of other people share your nervousness, and lines can be long before the race.

Lastly, if you take part in a road race, there are all kinds of goodies to be had. First and foremost, you'll most likely receive a commemorative T-shirt from the big event—a fairly equal trade for your ten- or twenty-dollar entry fee. Most races also have tables set up beyond the finish line with apples, bananas, PowerBars, soda, granola bars. Or sometimes they just hand you a bag full of free stuff from the sponsors—magazines, pens, key chains, samples of makeup and so on.

What to Expect in a Race

RACING IS AS SIMPLE AS . . .

- Register
- Pick up your bib and T-shirt
- Warm up and stretch
- Line up with your pace group
- Run the race!
- Cross the finish line
- Enjoy the free fruit, drinks and other goodies
- Cool down
- Feel proud of your participation!

I tend to be a pretty steady runner, so in a race, I keep the same pace at the end as in the beginning. I tend to find my groove pretty quickly.
Emily, 30

You can register for most races online or by fax prior to the race date. Or, if you decide at the last minute to run or you've been too busy to preregister, most races will allow you to sign up the morning of the event, except for large races like big-city marathons. After you're registered, you'll be able to pick up your number (these are called bibs) and a T-shirt. For most races you can just show up an hour (or less) before the race and go to the sign-in table, where you'll give them your name and in return you'll get a little paper bib with a number printed on it. Grab some safety pins and pin the number onto your top. Make sure and pin it to the shirt you think you'll be running in (in case you're wearing extra layers to stay warm before you run). Some races provide runners with "chips" in addition to bibs. These little electronic devices hook on to your shoelace, and they automatically register your time when you cross the finishing line. You'll need to return the chip at the end of the race.

If you've got a gym bag with your belongings, or you want to take off some of your layers of clothes before the race, many races will have a baggage area where you can leave your things with an attendant. At races sponsored by the New York Road Runners Club, they block off an area and separate it into groups marked 0 through 9. Then you put your bags in the pile that corresponds with the last number of your running bib. I've also seen people create some pretty inventive storage spaces for their belongings, including on tree branches, perched on top of a boulder and so on. There is an awful lot of trust among runners and the running community, and I've never heard of anyone's things disappearing during a race. While of course anything can happen, I guess the best rule of thumb is to use your own judgment.

After you've dropped off your belongings, take the time to warm up and stretch. Your warm-up is important before a race because most likely you'll be running faster than your normal running pace, if for no other reason than extra adrenaline and the spirit of the crowd. A good warm-up will give your heart and muscles a chance to get ready for the race, and will make your first mile of the race smoother. I usually jog anywhere between a half-mile and a mile as a prerace warm-up, depending on the distance of the race.

I warm up for a race the same way I do on other days, but I spend more time stretching each muscle.
Dayla, 26

It's usually around this time that I get struck with some prerace jitters, which usually leads me to the long line at the toilet. There I join everyone else suffering from prerace jitters. This is normal—all part of the body's way of letting us know that it's aware of what's going on. I often get stomach cramps and feel a strong urge to go to the bathroom before a race. This symptom generally goes away as soon as the race begins.

Follow the masses to find out where the start line is. Depending on how big the race is and how many runners are taking part, there may be "pace markers" set up behind the start line. These big numbered markers will be posted alongside the road, separated by anywhere from twenty to a hundred feet, again, depending on the number of runners. They'll most likely start at "6" and end at "10" or "12." These pace markers represent mile paces. Technically, only runners who plan to start and run the race at a six-minute mile pace should be standing in the area marked with a big "6," and so on down the line. I say technically, because it rarely works out this way. There's something about a starting line that makes many people, sometimes even those who are planning to walk the entire distance, feel the need to get as close to the front as they can. All I can say is, do this at your own risk. The faster runners can be pushy in getting out first, and sometimes there's a bit of elbowing that goes on at the beginning of a race as the faster runners try to break free of the pack. Just be aware that if you want to hang out near the start line and you're not planning on taking off at a fast clip, you may be bumped around a little bit. I recommend being realistic about your pace and line up with your marked group. Everyone will be happier for it.

I love racing! I think it's because I'm competitive in nature, and it's such a great test of my mental and physical strength. It's just you and your body out there, and it's awesome.
Laurie, 31

Depending on how big of an event the race is, there may be a person on a PA system walking you through some warm-ups and stretches, or telling you information about the race and its sponsors. I usually get in line for the race about 10 to 15 minutes before it starts, just so I can kind of find my spot in the lineup and chill out until it starts.

Starts for road races are a little different than starts for races around a track. The old "On your mark, get set . . . BANG" is what most people think of about the start of a race. Road races are a little different. They start with what's called a two command . . . "Runners to your marks . . . [pause]. . . . HONK!" The honk here represents an air horn.

And then you're off. If the race is crowded, be prepared to stand still for a minute (or more) and walk across the start line until the pack starts to thin out a bit and people can spread out and begin to run. The more crowded the race, the slower the start. If you want to mark your time for the race, take note of what the race clock says as you cross the starting line. You'll want to subtract this number from your finishing time to get a real representation of your race time. If it's a few seconds, you might not think it's a big deal, but depending on the size of the race and how far back you are, it could be a matter of minutes. In my first marathon, I had to take off over seven minutes from my finishing time . . . it took me that long just to get across the start. The top runners were well into their second mile by that time! If you're running in a race where the officials hand out timing chips, you won't have to worry about the starting lag. The chip will automatically record when you cross the start line, and give you an accurate race time when you've finished.

And now comes the fun part . . . run! You may find it takes you about a half-mile to find your own space, and your own pace. Keep in mind that whether you're trying to break a personal record or just want to finish the race, adrenaline will come into play. And adrenaline can be a great thing to help you through the race, and push you through to finish. But it can also nudge you to take off faster than you might have expected, or intended. I have done this so many times, and have suffered the consequences by being burned out halfway through the race. But even knowing this, I still find myself having to hold myself back during the first mile of any race. It's hard to get into a pace with runners all around, all running at different speeds. And it may seem like everyone's passing you, and fear of being the last one to come across the finish line will creep up. So you'll speed up, not wanting to be left behind. But it's always easier (and better) to start off slower and speed up once you're warmed up.

I'm only a ten-minute miler. I'll probably never be faster, but I'll be out there when I'm 80 years old. And that's my goal.
Sue, 55

I've been running road races for years, and I used to be very precise about it. I would set a goal of what speed I wanted to run the distance in, figure out a "per mile" pace, and then make myself hit that mark right from the start. The result? I often burned myself out in the first mile or two, and was so tired at the end that I inevitably slowed down, sometimes struggling even to finish. Then before a Corporate Challenge race in 1997, I asked a relatively fast woman on my team what her strategy was. She said that she usually started out slowly and then as her body warmed up, she sped up. Sounds simple, I know. So I tried it. It works. I still use this technique today—I even practice it during my regular runs. The only pitfall I run into when running like this is that sometimes I have all sorts of energy left over at the end of a race and I don't get to use it all up. This means that I could have run the whole race a little bit faster. But, again, it depends on what your goals are during a race—finish and feel good about it, or push yourself and run your fastest time.

During the race, take advantage of the water stations along the route, especially it it's hot or humid. As you approach the stations, expect a runner's traffic jam, and move to the outside of the route if you're not planning to stop. If you want to grab a cup of water, slow down and swoop a cup off of the table or from someone's extended hand. Staying well-hydrated during a race will make the whole experience a better one for you, and a couple of stops for water will ultimately add only a few seconds onto your finishing time. The art of running and drinking simultaneously is a difficult one. I still tend to slow down to a fast walk to guzzle down my cup or two. Otherwise I get all sorts of air in my belly and I can expect to amuse (or annoy) my fellow runners with some hearty belches throughout the next mile. A technique that does work well if you want to run and drink at the same time is the "fold and sip" technique. Generally, water cups at races are light paper cups that can easily be folded in half along the top. Now you've created a pointy spout that you can use to pour the water into your mouth as you continue running. When you're finished drinking, toss the cup in a trashcan or along the side of the road. If you've still got water in your cup when you're discarding it, lean down and gently set it down on the road—this way you won't splash water all over other runners' feet.

Many road race routes include a turnaround at some point, which means that the faster runners will be running toward you on the other side of the road. I love races with turnarounds because it gives me a chance to see the top runners and cheer for the top women. It's also a great distraction if you know people in the race. I get completely preoccupied looking for friends to yell for, which is great because I don't fixate on my own running and any discomfort I might be feeling.

My all-time favorite race was a 10K that I did in Waikiki, and we went around Diamond Head. What made it my favorite race was that all of the prizes were done by drawings. This gave it a noncompetitive flavor.
Paulette, 50

As you continue through the course, keep running and hang in there. Races will push you in more ways than you could imagine, no matter what your goals are. You will feel challenged. You will feel tired. And you will most definitely be looking forward to your first visual of the finish line. So . . . hang in there. It will be worth it, I promise. Slow down or speed up, depending on how you feel. And if you have to walk, walk. And if you can start running again in a little bit, go right ahead.

As you spy the finish line, you might find that people "kick" to the finish. This means that they sprint the last hundred meters or so, blowing by people, maybe even yourself, to reach the finish line. Derin gets annoyed when people kick at the end of a race and edge past him in the last few yards. It doesn't really bother me. I kick sometimes, too, but not to beat anybody else out. Only to try to get the fastest time I can for the race. And if I've got energy left at the end, why not? See how you feel. I usually find myself inspired at the end of a race . . . there are people standing along the side cheering for the runners, the clock over the finish line is ticking away, and I know my test of endurance is just about to end. I get a burst of energy, and I open up my stride a bit and pour it on a little. And it always feels great. To cross the finish line feeling strong gives me such a rush. I feel like my whole body is working together, like my arms and legs and hands and shoulders and hips have all been choreographed to perform the running dance. Sometimes there will be music (always upbeat) blasting over a loudspeaker near the finish line, too. This doesn't hurt. So finish strong, and cross the finish line feeling proud of yourself for what you've just accomplished.

I kick at the end of a race, definitely. In a race, it's amazing how I can just run so much faster and really push it at the end.
Bridget, 32

Once you cross the finish line, if your race is being officially timed (there are a fair number of "fun runs" that

> It's no surprise that women aren't as fast as men. On average, the top men are about 10 percent faster than the top women in a long-distance race.

don't keep official records of everyone's times), you'll be ushered into "chutes" or separate single-file lanes. Unless you're using the electronic timing chip, you'll have a little tag on your number bib that can be torn off. This will contain your number, age and sex. Rip this off, and hand it to the race official at the end of the chute. Voila. You're done. Congratulations! Beyond the finish line, you'll usually find water tables, boxes with fruit and all those goodies I talked about earlier. If you don't want to go home and crawl into bed, or leave straightaway to get brunch, hang around and watch the award ceremony. Race officials usually award prizes to the top three finishers in every age and gender group. Sometimes they have raffles. It's nice to kind of soak in the running culture after a race . . . you'll really feel the power of this community, and you're a part of it.

If your race was an official race for time (and not a fun run), you'll be able to find out exactly how you did, usually on a website associated with the race organizers. All you need is your bib number or your last name, and you'll be able to find out some vital statistics from the run. Here's an example of what statistics for a race would entail. These are my results from the Central California Half-Marathon in November 2000:

Total Ranking	Name	Age	Ranking among other women runners	Ranking among other women in age group	Finishing Time	Mile Pace
274	REBER	31	88/140	17/24	2:18:54	10:37

Why Race?

So, after that detailed description of what road races are like, aren't you a little more interested in taking a shot at it? Well, if you still need a little more convincing, you may be curious to know the answer to that big question . . . why race? Well, I can tell you one thing for sure. Most women who are taking part in the hundreds of road races that are held across the country every weekend are not doing it to win. They're doing it for the challenge. For the camaraderie. For all of the above.

Setting and Achieving Goals

I think what's exciting about racing is seeing people of all ages and stages of life coming out and having a good time and not necessarily being competitive. Races are very inclusive.
Gail, 52

I'm a very goal-oriented person. Meaning, I thrive on setting attainable goals for myself and then working to achieve them. I've realized that running is a perfect discipline for me because it easily fits into my strategy for getting through life. But even if you're not someone who moves forward by setting goals, try it for running, and see if it works for you. In the chapter on motivation, I talk about signing up for races as a way to keep running. But the very act of setting your sights on a race a month or two down the road, and then actually completing it, gives you a feeling you can't really put a label on.

My friend Alice started running at the age of thirty-two, and would often talk to me about running. It was really great to be a part of her progress. I had just moved to Los Angeles, and Alice told me she wanted to sign up for her first race—the Revlon 5K Run/Walk for Women, a national women's race held in New

York and Los Angeles to benefit women's cancer causes. She wanted to know if I thought she could do it, and I told her of course she could do it! I gave Alice a rough "training program" for the weeks leading up to the race so she'd feel confident about finishing and running the whole thing. She called me from her cell phone as soon as she finished the race and retrieved her things. I told her it was six in the morning, reminding her of the three-hour time difference. But I groggily listened to her shining on the other end. She was so happy and excited and surprised at herself. It was probably the best wake-up call I've ever gotten.

Personal Records

You might hear runners talk about running a PR. They're not talking about their fond memories of Puerto Rico. Most likely they're referring to a "personal record," which is exactly that. It's your personal fastest time running any particular distance. The great thing about PRs is, all you have to do is run one race, and you've instantly got one. And now that you've got one, you've got a time to beat. I have never run a road race as an adult where I was running against anything other than my own PR. Lord knows I'm not expecting to place in any of them. But knowing what my personal best times are at all of the different race distances gives me something to measure my time against. It's a good way to show me what kind of shape I'm in at any given time, and it's also a good motivator. But the best thing about personal records is that they're *personal*. It's between you, yourself and you. And when you set a new PR

I'm not out there racing to finish in the top hundred. I'm out there to have fun, to cross the finish line, to have that sense of accomplishment. I feel like a kid in a candy store because it's something that's so new to me.
Karen, 29

I'm pretty competitive with myself, so every time I go out and run a race, I try to beat my time before. I also compete with other women out there running, but it's more of a game that I play to get myself to run faster.
Bridget, 32

during a race, even if it's by a few seconds, it's a great feeling of accomplishment.

One spring about four years ago, I set new PRs in a bunch of different distances. I was unstoppable. Granted, this was the spring after my nasty breakup, and I was in damn good shape (I had to do something with all of that anxious energy). It was pretty cool though. After running races for about three or four years, I was suddenly running faster then ever. Today those are still the personal records I try to top in every race. I haven't done it yet. But I'm not finished trying.

I like just being around other runners but still doing it for myself. I love that adrenaline thing.
Alice, 34

Camaraderie

One of the greatest things about the races themselves for me is seeing how many runners participate. It never ceases to amaze me how many people have made the effort to get up so early, freeze their butts off on a cold winter morning and gleefully submit themselves to a strange form of torture. It's really inspiring. And the best part is, runners, as a community, are really great people. Perhaps it's the shared nervousness and the prerace jitters that bring everyone together—I don't know. But runners actually talk to each other before races, share jokes, bad stories about past races, complain about the late start. And frankly, these days it's hard to feel like a part of a community or group in most cities. For many of us, our workplace constitutes the extent of our social circle. That and a few friends from college or the neighborhood. But runners instantly accept other runners . . . I swear. It's an interesting phenomenon.

I ran a 10K race during the spring when I was running so

strong, and was feeling really good for most of the race. With about two miles to go, a woman running next to me complimented me on my running top. I was sporting a colorful red, orange and black tie-dyed top that had been designed by a friend. I thanked the woman and told her the story behind the top, and we kept running, side-by-side. By this point, I was starting to run out of steam. But we continued to talk and supported each other through the rest of the race, crossing the finish line at the same time. I ran my fastest 10K that day, and I honestly don't think I could have done it without that woman. I have no idea who she is, although I can still picture her in my head.

Women-Only Events and Races for a Cause

Still not convinced? In the past few years there has been a real surge in women's running, and likewise, in women's running events. Talk about inspirational. There's a national race you may have heard of called Race for the Cure, which is held in cities across the country every spring. Proceeds from the race go to help cure breast cancer, and it's a women-only event. Among the thousands and thousands of runners, many of them are wearing banners on the backs of their shirts. Some read "In Celebration of . . ." and then someone's name. Others read "In Memory of . . ." And so on. That event never fails to profoundly affect me. There is something so powerful about being part of a cause, of a movement that is filled with so much positive energy. I am never prouder to be a woman and a

Running for an organized run like Race for the Cure is great. It's more about getting involved in a cause, and you share more than just running with the people beside you.
AnneMarie, 32

runner than I am on days like that. The love and energy of the crowd is invigorating, and for the time it takes me to run that 5K distance, my purpose on this earth is suddenly very clear.

Women-only races are great, too, because we are the stars of the race! Women get to cross the finish line first! And many beginning women runners feel more comfortable running in women-only events because they're less self-conscious about how well they do and how they look doing it. To me, women-only races have a different vibe. And it's a vibe that I love.

There are many races, though, that aren't women-only events. But for me, there is nothing better than running for a cause. Talk about good karma! Running for causes like helping the homeless or funding AIDS and cancer research, truly makes a difference, both monetarily, and in your spirit, support and positive energy.

At the end of this chapter is a list of women-only national events, most of which fund-raise for various women's causes. I challenge you to find a race in your town and sign up for it. You won't regret it, I promise.

Running locked into a lifestyle after I ran my first race—the Avon 10K. It was just the most amazing experience, and that was what hooked me.
Christie, 29

Women-only racing is a great way to start, but more women today are running races than when I started 15 years ago.
Libby, 41

The Different Road Races

All right. If I've done my job right, you're convinced that road races aren't evil, and you may actually have an interest in participating in one someday soon. Now the question is, what kind of race should you run? Here is a look at a variety of road races.

2 Miles: While this isn't that common a racing distance, you may be able to find one near you. A two-mile race is a great distance to try out racing, because it's short enough that the pain is over quickly, but you'll still get the experience of racing. Many of these shorter runs are considered *fun runs*, meaning they don't keep formal times for the runners, and you might find that they accompany a longer event such as a 10K. My favorite two-mile race takes place in Central Park every January. It's called the Hot Chocolate Two-Miler. And all runners get free hot chocolate and bagels after the race. Short and sweet.

5K (3.1 miles): You've probably heard of a 5K before, and that's because this is the most common of the road racing distances. If you ever ran cross-country or knew someone who did, this is the traditional length of any cross-country course. This is my favorite distance to run, because it's long enough that you can't possibly be expected to run it all-out for the entire thing, and it's short enough that you can push yourself harder, knowing that it won't be too long before you're finished. The top elite runners run this event in 13:00 or under. My personal record is 23:51, and that usually lands me somewhere in the top third or half of the women runners. This distance is also great for beginning runners because if you find you want to walk some of the race, you'll still finish the race in under 50:00.

8K (approximately 5 miles): This is a relatively new racing distance, but 8K's are cropping up here and there. This is a good transition race between a 5K and a 10K.

10K (6.2 miles): The 10K is probably the second most common racing distance after the 5K. I used to dread this distance. It's fairly long if you're used to running three or four miles for your normal run, and I often found myself burned out by mile five with not much steam to get me through to the finish. But the 10K has grown on me a bit (it's still not my favorite). There are a

The first race I ran was the Cooper Bridge 10K, and when I got to the finish line I just wept. Here I was raising two kids, and this race was something I did totally for myself. Karen, 39

I love running the longer distances because it gives my body time to adjust and fit into a groove where running becomes rhythmic and comfortable.
Eileen, 26

lot of runners who love this distance because it's long enough for them to really find their pace and get into a groove. They can't do that as well during a 5K because they consider it too short.

Half Marathon (13.1 Miles): This is one distance I'm becoming very familiar with lately, as I'm using it as a training tool for the marathon. This is exactly half the distance of a marathon, and many of the runners you'll find here are in training for a longer event. Another distance I used to dread, I'm now a fan of the half-marathon. Running one is a very different experience than a 5K or even a 10K, because there's just so much more time to think about things. Like, "When is this damn race going to be over?" and so on. But it's those same moments of doubt and exhaustion that make the finish that much more rewarding. It's a sick game, but there are a lot of players.

I really like half-marathons because it pushes me, but I know it's going to end.
Maggie, 25

Marathon (26.2 miles): The ultimate race. Well, of course there are ultramarathons (50–100 miles), triathlons and other assorted craziness, but many consider the marathon to be the ultimate road race. Myself included. I do not run these fast, by any stretch of the imagination. I'm happy that I run the whole thing at all. But for those of you out there who wish you could run a marathon but don't think it's something your body is capable of doing, I'm here to prove you wrong. My body was built for short bursts of speed. I'm a sprinter. If I run over eight

You could lose your house, you could lose all the money in the world, but you can't lose the fact that you finished the race. That will be with you forever.
Lauren, 35

miles or so, my body's kind of like, "Whoa . . . what do you think you're doing?" and it slows down. And this is just fine with me. I don't aspire to be a fast marathon runner. Just to finish without killing myself. And as difficult as they are, running that first marathon was one of the most personally fulfilling things I've ever done in my life. I was on an emotional high for months. And if you're one of those women with a secret interest in conquering this beast, I say, "do it!"

Some Great Races for Women

Race for the Cure

The Komen Race for the Cure, which I mentioned earlier, is the largest all-women's race in the country. The year 2001 will be the eleventh year for the event, which has grown to include more than 100 different races held all over the U.S. One of the things that makes this race so fulfilling to participate in is that it's in support of such a great cause. Just by signing up and paying your entry fee, you're contributing to finding a cure for women's cancers, specifically breast cancer. It's a huge movement that seems to be gaining momentum every year. Two years ago in New York City, they even added a component for the men in your lives to participate. For a separate entrance fee, your husband, boyfriend, brother, or friend can have his own T-shirt and baseball hat and be steered in the direction of different preplanned men's cheering sections. Derin wasn't so sure when I first signed him up, but he wore his T-shirt with pride, and it was nice to know he was there when I rounded the corner at mile two. In 1998, the Race for the Cure raised over $1 million in grants to directly support research and resources pertaining to women and cancer. Go to *www.raceforthecure.com* for information and a schedule of races near you.

I ran in a race that was for women's cancers, and the camaraderie was amazing. You wouldn't think you'd have that experience in a race.
Sarah, 26

Did you know that 1972 was the first year women were allowed to run in the Boston Marathon (the country's oldest)?

Avon Running

Avon (yes, the beauty products company) has a Running Global Women's Circuit, and they've been involved in supporting women-only running events since the 1970s. In fact, Avon was heavily involved in the fight to get the women's marathon added as an event in the Olympics, the first of which was held in the 1984 Summer Olympics. According to their website, the goal of their running program is to "encourage women worldwide to the starting line of fitness through grassroots events so they can experience the positive rewards of a regular running or walking regimen." And it seems to be working. Today, Avon's Running Global Women's Circuit sponsors races across the country, usually in the form of the "Avon Mini-Marathon," a 10K race. For more information on this event, check out their website at *www.avoncompany.com/women/avonrunning/*.

RRCA Women's Distance Festival

This festival was launched by the Road Runners Club of America in 1979 to bring attention to the fact that there weren't as many women's distance running events in the Olympics as men's. But even now that women are on equal footing (pun intended) with men regarding the Olympic events, the Festival continues to grow as a way to celebrate women's running in general. They focus on "low-key," nonintimidating events like 5Ks or walking events, and part of the program is designed specifically to support the beginning woman runner! Events are held in over 29 states across the country, and they generally take place over the summer. For a schedule of events by state, check out the RRCA's website at *www.rrca.org/events*.

Revlon 5K Run/Walk for Women

This race, which is the only one mentioned here that allows the participation of men, started in 1993 to raise money for women's cancer programs. Currently, there are only events in Los Angeles and New York, but they are big events to be sure. In just those two cities in 1999, more than 100,000 people came out to support the event, including Revlon spokesmodels Cindy Crawford and Melanie Griffith. It was nice to see such a diverse group of people supporting this cause. And, the goody bags at the end had all kinds of makeup samples from Revlon. *www.revlonrunwalk.com*.

So, what do you say? Think you might be interested in giving it a try? Go for it! I guarantee you'll experience some of the wonderful benefits of running a race, and you'll be proud of yourself for taking the chance.

I commit to signing up for and running one road race in the next six months.

Signed _____

Date _____

11.

Want to Pick up the Pace?

Getting Stronger, Getting Faster

The primary goal of speed workouts, as you might have guessed by now, is to build speed in your body and enable you to run distances faster. They're a great way to build speed if you're training for a particular distance race like the 5K. But even if this isn't your goal, do me a favor and keep reading. Speed workouts have other benefits that may make them a welcome part of your workout. For one thing, even though speed training consists of some form of running or another, it really provides your body with a whole new type of workout. Most speed training really results in building muscle, which is something your regular runs won't do to a large extent. Secondly, speed training is a nice break from the same old run day in and day out. Depending on what type of speed workout you want to do, it may take you half the time of your usual workout to complete. And it gives you a chance to flex new muscles, literally and figuratively.

When I ran the intermediate hurdles in high school and college, my teammates and I dreaded speed workouts. Well, come to think of it, pretty much all of our track workouts could be considered speed workouts. When I switched to running longer distances, I thought my days of timed laps around the track were over. But in the past few years, I've built speed training back into my workouts, along with weight training and yoga, and found my body responded very well. Not only did cross-training help strengthen those muscles that running wasn't really reaching, it also made a big difference in my long distance race pace.

Speed Training

I have had the pleasure (or pain, depending on how you look at it) of doing speed workouts in some form or another since sixth grade when I first started running track. Since then, I've gone through a handful of coaches in middle school, high school, college and even in New York when I ran with the UN Running Club. The speed workouts below are a compilation of the many I've done over the past (nineteen!) years.

What I hate about speed workouts is that I know how important they are and I don't do them. They're hard!
AnneMarie, 32

Interval Training

Interval training is one of the most popular forms of speed training. It involves running certain distances multiple times in a workout, with a rest in between each run. For example, if you want to do mile intervals, you would run your miles one at a time, stopping in between each one to allow your heart rate to

I used to do speed workouts when I was in college—we'd do uphill sprints and stadium stairs. Now I just focus on distance running.
Emily, 30

return to normal. The goal in doing interval work is that because you're allowing your body to rest in between each interval, you can push yourself while you're running to go a little faster than you would if you were stringing all of the miles together.

For example, if I were going to do mile intervals, I would first pick the number of miles I wanted to run. I usually do mile intervals on a track, and in groups of three. When I run three miles consecutively, I might run them in a total time of twenty-six or twenty-seven minutes, or an average of eight and a half to nine minutes per mile. But when I'm doing mile intervals, I might push myself to run each individual mile in seven minutes. Because I know I can stop after each mile and cool down for several minutes, I'm willing to push my body harder in anticipation of the pending relief.

You can do intervals at any distance, or you can use running time as a measurement instead of actual distance. One of my most grueling interval workouts was at Penn State, where the head coach Teri Jordan had us running ten four-hundred-meter (quarter mile) intervals, with two minutes in between. That two minutes in between had to be spent doing situps or jumping jacks or some other high-intensity exercise. Interval workouts like that could cause a girl to throw up. And they often did. I'm not saying you should do these kinds of speed workouts. Although sometimes I do a variation of this workout around the track at the high school around the corner. My variation includes a lot fewer intervals, and I actually enjoy it.

While many interval workouts are run on a track because the distances are so clearly marked, you can make up workouts anywhere you run. You can choose to run in four-block intervals, or loops around a park. Whatever makes the most sense for you, give it a try. Here is a sampling of some interval workouts I do when trying to improve my speed on a middle-distance race like the 5K. Again, with regards to the speed that you do these workouts, I would only encourage you to run them at a pace that is faster than your usual run, as opposed to sprinting, so you can get your body used to going at a quicker pace. The idea is, if you can train at a seven-minute mile pace for three one-mile intervals, eventually you'll be able to run the entire distance strung together at the same pace.

Take what you want from these workouts and make them work for you! Don't forget to recover in between each interval for anywhere from two to five minutes. I generally walk one lap around the track in between each interval to fully recover.

SAMPLE INTERVAL WORKOUT #1

- 2 × 1 mile (four laps around track) with rest in between each mile, followed by

- 2 × 800 meters (half-mile or two laps around track) with rest in between each 800 meters

SAMPLE INTERVAL WORKOUT #2:

- 4 × 800 meters (half-mile or two laps around track) with rest in between each 800 meters

SAMPLE INTERVAL WORKOUT #3:

- 6 × 400 meters (quarter-mile or one lap around track) with rest in between each 400 meters

SAMPLE INTERVAL WORKOUT #4:

- 2 × 1 mile (four laps around track) with rest in between each mile, followed by

- 2 × 800 meters (half-mile or two laps around track) with rest in between each 800 meters, followed by

- 4 × 400 meters (quarter-mile or one lap around track) with rest in between each 400 meters

Fartleks

This name is always bound to raise eyebrows. Anyway, fartlek is a real, bonafide term among the running community, and it's a type of speed workout that was designed by Gosta Holmer, a Swedish Olympic track coach, to give his athletes a variation on traditional interval workouts.

I find fartleks are easier on a treadmill. If I did them outside, I wouldn't know how fast I was going. I do timed intervals and hit my pace perfectly on a treadmill.
Alice, 34

While fartleks are very similar to intervals in that they include bursts of speed at distances shorter than you typically run, the difference with fartleks is that you don't ever stop running. Here's an example of one of my typical fartlek workouts to show you how it works. If I'm doing my four-mile loop, I would set out at a slow pace—generally slower than my usual run, focusing on staying relaxed. About four minutes into my run, I turn up the speed and push myself at race pace for the next four minutes. Once these four minutes are up, I revert back to my slower jogging pace for the next four minutes, and so on.

Fartleks are a great workout because they ensure that you're still getting all of the distance in of a regular run, but you're getting the benefits of a full-fledged speed workout on top of that.

They are an excellent way to build up speed and endurance. They can be very intense, depending on which variables you choose for your hard and easy running periods. I usually do fartlek workouts as the last workout prior to a particular race, and always for a distance that's a little longer than the race I'm training for. So, a four-mile fartlek is a great speed workout for a 5K, which is only 3.1 miles. The goal here is that I'll be able to push myself for longer periods of time in the race because I'll be accustomed to pushing my body at a point where it's already exhausted. And fartleks can be extremely exhausting. Usually by the last couple of intense bursts, I have to walk for a minute before starting up into my jog to allow myself time to recover.

Here are some sample fartlek workouts that you can borrow from to make a workout that works for you:

SAMPLE FARTLEK WORKOUT #1:

- Jog for four minutes, run hard for one minute. Repeat for entire distance of run.

SAMPLE FARTLEK WORKOUT #2:

- Jog for four minutes, run hard for four minutes. Repeat for entire distance of run

SAMPLE FARTLEK WORKOUT #3:

- Walk for two minutes, jog for three minutes, run hard for five minutes. Repeat for entire distance of run.

Hill Workouts

Hill workouts used to be my favorite type of speed workout. Don't ask me why. I guess in a lot of ways I'm a glutton for punishment. Actually, I think it comes from my history as a sprinter. My body is always happier running short bursts of speed than long, slow distances. So, when I'm doing hill workouts, I really feel my whole body working together, and I can imagine that my hamstrings and quadriceps are getting stronger with every step.

I love hills. I think they make you really strong, so I incorporate them into my run.
Janet, 51

Don't get me wrong. As much as I love hill workouts, I hate them, too. They are among the most painful of speed workouts, that is, if you're doing them right. Each hill that you run should wear you out to the point of exhaustion . . . to the point that you couldn't go another step farther. That's when you're really doing your body some good.

In the world of running, there are two kinds of hills: sprinter's hills and distance runner's hills. Sprinter's hills are characterized by being relatively steep and short. By short, I mean around one-to-two-hundred meters long (under a quarter-mile). Distance runner's hills on the other hand, are generally not very steep, in fact, sometimes you don't even realize there's a gradient there until you reach the top and look behind you. These hills are also generally much longer in length (a half-mile or longer).

When doing hill workouts, most people tend to focus on the sprinter's hills, and pick a number of times they plan to push themselves up the hill. The goal in running these hills is to run them at about eighty to ninety percent of your top speed. So, not an all-out sprint (or you wouldn't have the energy to do more than one), but very intense nonetheless. You should feel a slight burning in your thighs as you strive to reach the end marker. Take a rest in between each hill to allow yourself to recover by walking back downhill.

Hill workouts provide really great opportunities, not only to strengthen your muscles, but to strengthen your stride as well. The longer your stride is on your way up the hill, the harder your leg muscles have to work with each step to propel you forward at top speed. When you do these, focus on your stride and think about your form with every step you take. Feel the power in your legs and arms and torso as you push yourself onward. Use your arms to get you where you're going—arms are invaluable in helping you get up hills.

Mixing It Up

Speed workouts can be a great addition to your running program, but they shouldn't replace all of your runs. Ideally, you don't want to do more than one or two speed workouts a week, and you'll want to avoid doing speed workouts two days in a row. They are meant to compliment your training, but not dominate it.

You'll also see benefits by incorporating a weekly long run into your schedule. In running terms, this is called LSD, or *long slow distance*. This weekly run is more about the amount of time you run as opposed to the actual distance covered, so your speed isn't important. LSD is a staple of marathon training, but beyond that, it's a great way to teach your body about

Once a week I do speed work with a coach and about 15 runners. There's great camaraderie and we're pretty competitive—no one wants to be the last one to finish during our sets of repeats. Eileen, 26

endurance. I usually do my long, slow runs on Sundays, when I've got plenty of time and I can enjoy the run. Again—run this as slow as you like. The idea is not to run farther distances, but to lengthen the workout itself. When you're doing a long run, make sure you're properly hydrated, and bring along some water or even a gel or sports drink. These will help fuel your body throughout the run.

Here are some examples of how you might incorporate speed and distance into your running schedule:

EXAMPLE #1:

Monday	OFF
Tuesday	Standard Run
Wednesday	OFF
Thursday	Standard Run
Friday	Fartlek
Saturday	OFF
Sunday	Long Slow Distance

EXAMPLE #2:

Monday	OFF
Tuesday	Standard Run
Wednesday	Fartlek
Thursday	Standard Run
Friday	OFF
Saturday	Standard Run
Sunday	Long Slow Distance

EXAMPLE #3:

Monday	Standard Run
Tuesday	Interval Training
Wednesday	OFF
Thursday	Standard Run
Friday	Hill Workout
Saturday	Standard Run (or shorter than usual)
Sunday	Long Slow Distance

Cross-Training

Just as the key to good nutrition and a healthy lifestyle is balance, so it is with staying physically fit. It's important to include other types of activities in your life. While running is a great cardiovascular exercise, it doesn't work every muscle in your body. And not doing any activity outside of running can eventually lead to boredom, which can lead to dropping the sport altogether.

I try to continue participating in a variety of different activities in my life to compliment my running. I always have. My alternative activities vary, depending on what's going on in my life, what resources I have access to or what season it is. A few years ago, I went through an aerobics phase, both body sculpting and step aerobics. I did two to three classes a week on my lunch break at work, and I found it to be a great way to work out my upper body and strengthen my muscles. Since moving to Southern California, I've gotten into hiking, in-line skating,

I think it's really important to shake it up and do all sorts of different things so your body doesn't get too used to any one thing. I do weights, kickboxing and modern dance. Amy, 30

tennis and of course, yoga. Regardless of what you do on the side, alternative workouts are a great way to add variety to your day, and keep you healthy and strong. Here are some exercise options that are especially complimentary to running.

Weight Training

Weight training is probably one of the most important cross-training exercises you can do. Unless you're doing those speed workouts mentioned previously in this chapter, you're not building much muscle when you run. And it's a known fact that the higher our muscle to fat ratio, the more efficiently our bodies will function. So building and maintaining muscle mass is pretty important stuff.

Whereas I used to belong to a gym where I could workout with weights on my lunch break a few times a week, I haven't rejoined a gym since we moved. Instead, Derin and I bought some simple hand weights at a sporting goods store, and we do weights together. In fact, I'll even admit that I "host" a body-sculpting class in our living room every now and then, which basically means I preprogram a bunch of CD's to play aerobic-type music and then Derin and I do our workout, with me calling out what to do. It's kind of a joke and we laugh for much of the workout because I generally spaz out and dive into the role of aerobics instructor, but we still get the workout in. Our weight-lifting workouts tend to consist of the following types of exercises:

- Bicep curls
- Triceps extensions

I've started doing some upper body weight training, figuring I would be a better runner. I'm more aware of my body and my arms now.
Sue, 55

I teach physical education, so I consider that my cross-training!
Karen, 25

- Squats
- Leg lifts
- Situps
- Pushups

Yoga

Yoga is a great complement to running, because it is about stretching and breathing and is completely low impact. "Yoga" means union, and in the western version of yoga, it generally involves a combination of physical poses, breathing exercises and meditation. All three of these elements are invaluable in helping us relieve stress in our everyday lives and do something truly healing for our body. The poses also offer opportunity for great stretches, which can only help in preventing running injuries and keep us feeling loose, limber and strong.

I've become completely hooked on yoga. I think it's a really good way of counter-balancing the shortening of muscles and repetitive motion of running.
Beth, 35

Hiking

You don't have to trek up Mount Kilimanjaro to get a good workout in. Hiking to any degree is a great thing. Derin and I hike with our dog, Ari, at a place called Runyon Canyon in Los Angeles. The hour-long hike up and down the canyon is enough to get all three of our heart rates up, and rewards us with a great view of Los Angeles when we reach the top (when there's no smog, that is). Hiking is something we often do with our nonrunning friends, too, so it provides a way to socialize while still doing something healthy and physically active.

Swimming

Many runners who choose not to run outdoors year round because of cold weather opt to swim in the winters instead. Swimming is an excellent cardiovascular activity, and it's completely no-impact, so it's ideal for people coming off of injuries or runners who want to give their legs a break. My friend Alice is currently in the midst of a cold New York City winter and signed up with a water running class through the New York Road Runners Club. Once a week, she meets her class at a swimming pool, and they do their entire running workout in the water! I haven't tried this yet, but Alice is addicted. And when spring hits New York and she laces up her shoes to hit the park, she'll be even stronger than she was when she left off in the park.

In-Line Skating

Shortly after I moved to Los Angeles, I bought a new pair of Rollerblades. I had an old pair in New York, but the steep downhills in Central Park scared the crap out of me, so I never went skating beyond the flat part, which doesn't amount to very much. But now I have the Strand to skate on—a long cement path running parallel to the ocean, starting in Santa Monica and running down below Hermosa and Redondo beaches.

While we don't do this regularly, every now and then Derin and I will drag our neighbors to Santa Monica to Rollerblade up and down the Strand. And let me tell you something—it is hard work. Even on a flat surface, I'm feeling muscles I never even knew existed. By the time I've finished, my inner and outer thighs are sore, and my calves are tight. In-line skating is also great because it provides you with a low-impact alternative to running.

Biking

In interviewing women for this book, I found that many supplemented their running with biking, either long distance or mountain biking. Perhaps that's because biking is very similar to running in that it can be a solo activity. Biking intensely focuses on the leg muscles, especially the quadriceps. Biking is also great if you're considering doing any sort of triathlon down the road.

When I lived in Seattle I used to mountain bike after work for an hour or two. And it's really hilly there, so I'd get a great workout. My legs would get real strong, and my arms, too.

Bridget, 32

Boxing

Boxing is one of my favorite workouts. Aside from running, of course. Boxing and kickboxing are starting to become very popular, thanks in part to Billy Blanks's Tae Bo phenomenon. I took a boxing class for about a year with my best friend, AnneMarie, and we had a blast hitting the punching bag, doing shadow boxing, using the focus pads. Boxing is an intense workout because the idea behind it is you're always on the go. You're always jumping rope, or punching the bag or doing something that results in an outpouring of sweat and raised heart rate.

Cross-training is important because it prevents boredom. It also helps train your body more thoroughly and more effectively for any sport you are doing.

Gail, 52

Whatever your goals are in the beginning of a running program, you'll surely see the rewards of your running in your other activities. And visa versa. Any cross-training you take on will absolutely make you a stronger runner and a well-rounded, fit woman.

Epilogue:
The Cool Down

Congratulations! If you're reading this page, hopefully you've made a commitment to make running a part of your life. You've tried it a few times. And you even kind of like it. And now that you're in on all the "secrets," you've pledged to become a full-time member of the running society.

As you put this book down and go on with your busy life, there will be many things that come along to do their best to keep you from running. There will be crunch times at work, holidays, family obligations, sickness, weather. You name it, it can become an obstacle in your path. But now you know all the detours. A little planning, a running date here and there and flexibility will get you through the hard times. And they'll make the good runs feel all that much better. So, become a part of a national movement in women's health and empowerment—keep running! Experience and enjoy the many rewards that a running lifestyle can give you. I hope to see you out there on the road!

Debbie

Acknowledgments

Wow. An acknowledgments page. I've never had to do one of these before, and so many people have helped and inspired me along the way. I hope I don't forget anyone! To my husband, Derin, who watched this idea evolve from a bunch of scraps of paper written while watching Ari play at the dog run to this book. You've given me the support, patience, energy and peace of mind to write this book, and I thank you for your never-ending love, and for your invaluable input. You are my rock. My parents, Dale and MaryLou, the most wonderful parents a girl could ask for. I can still hear your voices yelling for me when you came to my high school track meets to cheer me on. Thank you for encouraging me to run and supporting my writing and running habits. My sister, Michele, whose illustrations grace the pages of this book—thank you for taking the time out of your hectic schedule to contribute. Watching you blossom into a runner over the past year has been incredibly inspirational to me. I hope we get to run together one day! My in-laws, Barbara and David Basden, and my outlaws, Leslie Basden, Angie Welton and Lynn Welton—thank you for welcoming me to California and for being so supportive of my writing, which undoubtedly eats up a lot of my free weekends.

To everyone who read my first proposal, including Shantha Bloemen, Claire Curley, Sarah Landy and my mom-in-law, Barbara Basden—your feedback and thoughtful notes helped me fill in the gaps. To Christie Dreyfuss, my running partner, peer and friend (and you, too, Kevin!)—thanks for your support and encouragement throughout this whole process, and for listening to me babble during our early morning runs when you were still half-asleep. To Alice Wilder, whose own new running career has been an inspiration to watch—thanks for reading draft after draft and giving me such great perspective. To AnneMarie Kane, my best friend ever, who has been behind me at every stage of this process—thank you for your boundless support and your friendship. To Angela Santomero, who encouraged me to write my first published book—thank you for believing in me. To Loch Phillips and Lee Skaife, for your incredible friendship. I'm so happy to be a part of your lives. To Tip Blish and Bridget Perry, who made the move to California much easier by being such wonderful neighbors and running partners.

To Emily Caroline, thank you for your help in meeting such wonderful women runners in the Boston area, and for taking the time to read a (very) rough draft of this book. And to all of the women who opened up and shared their personal running experiences with me: Alfreda, Colleen Banse, Libby Bishop, Laura Brown, Laurie Bruce-Rech, Shareena Carlson, Emily Caroline, Lauren Cepeda, Dayla Corcoran, Christie Dreyfuss, Gail Edie, Beth Gerber, Maggie Haines, Janet Hale, Amy Handler, Karen Ivins, AnneMarie Kane, Sue Kaplan, Sarah Landy, Pamela Levine, Karen Linson, Eileen Magilligan, Naomi, Bridget Perry, Michele Reber, Robin Reid, Sarah Reines, Deena Weise, Karen Wester, Alice Wilder, Emily Voytek. Thank you for your frankness, your enthusiasm and your inspiration. A special thanks also to the Western Massachusetts Women's Running Club—I wish you the best of luck as you continue to grow!

To my agents, Susan Schulman and Christine Morin, who believed in the book enough to persevere and find the right publisher. You've been wonderful to work with, and I am grateful for your friendship. To Sheila Curry Oakes at Perigee Books, who saw what I was trying to do with *Run for Your Life*, and believed in it enough to take a chance with it. And to my editor, Jennifer Repo, thank you so much for all of the support and strength you brought to this project.

To Freddi Carlip and the RRCA—thank you for your continual support and enthusiasm for this project, and for the RRCA's strong commitment to women's running.

To Linda Simensky, my boss at Cartoon Network and my friend—thanks for your enthusiasm for this book, and for making writing it while working for you an easy task.

To my high school track coaches, the Reiders, Whitney Seltzer, Lance Atkins and Mr. Banker. You all were patient with my obsession with the hurdles and fostered a love of running in me that continues. To Teri Jordan, PSU Track Coach, for being so patient with my speed (or lack of it) and encouraging me onward. And to Jorge Hernandez-Mora, former head coach of the UN Track Club. You always treated me like a serious runner even though I wasn't the fastest on the team, and I will forever be grateful that you believed in me enough to put me on the Milrose Games Mile Relay. Your friendship, encouragement and coaching expertise played a key role in keeping me running through my hectic years in NYC. To my first running mentors, Sue Heinz and Jenny Russell, and my running partners along the way: Laurie Bruce, Carolyn Camburn, Jeanette Gonzalez and Frank Lourenso. You've all given me reason to run and I thank you!

Resources

Lioness: A clothing line designed as an answer for the dearth of women's running clothes on the market. The Lioness website offers a list of retailers where their clothing is available, as well as online ordering capability. *www.lionessrun.com*

Moving Comfort: The biggest name in women's fitness clothing made by women for women. Products are available in stores like REI, Nordstrom, and through Title 9 Sports catalogs. Moving Comfort also has a website that lists retailers that sell their clothes near you. 4500 Southgate Place, Suite 800, Chantilly, VA 20151-1729. Tel: 800-763-6000. *www.movingcomfort.com*

Rykä: Athletic and running shoes made specifically for women. 6 Clock Tower Place, Suite 100, Maynard, MA 01754. Tel: 888-834-RYKA. *www.ryka.com*

Title 9 Sports: Comprehensive catalog for women-only running and athletic apparel. Tel: 800-342-4448. *www.title9sports.com*

Two Roads Fitness: Specializes in clothing made to a woman's shape, maximizing function and great fit. 1440 Sheldon Street, St. Paul, MN 55208. Tel: 800-240-8176, 651-603-0954. *http://store.yahoo.com/trfitness/*

X-Chrom: Online catalog specializing in women's sport apparel, with a large athletic bra selection. 7181 W. Grand Avenue, Chicago, IL 60707. Tel: 773-385-9557. *www.x-chrom.com*

WEBSITES WITH RUNNING INFORMATION FOR WOMEN

Running Times: The online site for the traditional magazine, which includes a list of women-only races. *www.runningtimes.com*

Sports for Women: Creates original interactive content; aggregates the latest women's sports news, scores and statistics; and packages programming for distribution on the website. *www.sportsforwomen.com*

Women's Multisport OnLine: An online hub for women's sports, including running, triathlons, cycling and swimming. Includes an online bookstore, linked with Amazon. *www.womensmultisport.com*

Women's Running: General information on running for women, along with a complete list and calendar of women-only races (associated with *Runner's World* magazine) *www.womens-running.com/community/home.html*

Women's Sports Foundation: A charitable educational organization dedicated to increasing the participation of girls and women in sports and fitness and creating an educated public that supports gender equity in sport. *www.womenssportsfoundation.org*

GENERAL RUNNING AND FITNESS ORGANIZATIONS

American Council on Exercise: A nonprofit organization committed to promoting active, healthy lifestyles and their positive effects on the mind, body and spirit. *www.acefitness.org*

American Running Association: A nonprofit, educational association of runners, medical professionals and corporations dedicated to promoting running nationwide. 4405 East West Highway, Suite 405, Bethesda, MD 20814. Tel: 800-776-2732. *www.americanrunning.org*

National Association for Girls and Women in Sports: An organization that champions equal funding, quality and respect for women's sports programs. *www.aahperd.org/nagws/nagws_main.html*

RRCA (Road Runners Club of America): The Road Runners Club of America is a national organization of over 700 Chapter Clubs located in 48 states and Guam, and representing over 200,000 members. They are heavily involved in supporting women's running. 510 N. Washington Street, Alexandria, VA 22314. Tel: 703-836-0558. *www.rrca.org*

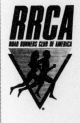

ON-LINE RUNNING HUBS

Active.com: This site boasts information on numerous sports, but specifically has a fantastic national calendar with road race schedules and online registration capability. *www.active.com*

Kicksports: The complete online resource for runners. Includes a great online training log and a service to find running partners around the country, based on pace and distance. *www.kicksports.com*

On the Run: Online resource for the long-distance running community. *www.ontherun.com*

Runner's Web: A running and triathlon resources site. *www.runnersweb.com*

Run the Planet: The largest running community on the Internet. Includes a searchable database of running routes and information on running throughout the world. *www.runtheplanet.com*

Runner's World magazine: A hub for the magazine, with a lot of helpful information, including an area specific to women and running. *www.runnersworld.com*

Avon Running: A series of international and national 10K and 5K races for women. *www.avoncompany.com/women/avonrunning/*

Revlon Run/Walk for Women: A growing race held in Los Angeles and New York, to fund women's cancer research. *www.revlonrunwalk.com*

RRCA Women's Distance Festival: Events are held in over 29 states across the country, and they generally take place over the summer. For a schedule of events by state, go to *www.rrca.org/events*

RUNNING TEAMS FOR NATIONAL CAUSES

National AIDS Marathon Training Program: A six-month physical-conditioning program geared to beginning and experienced runners that prepares participants to run a marathon while raising money for AIDS-related services. *www.aidsmarathon.com*

Team Diabetes: Organized by the American Diabetes Association, this marathon program includes training, workouts, monthly clinics and fund-raising support, all to benefit the Diabetes Association. *www.diabetes.org*

Team in Training: Organized by The Leukemia and Lymphoma Society, this training program includes training, schedules, coaching, clinics, travel and accommodations, and fund-raising support. All proceeds benefit The Leukemia and Lymphoma Society. *www.teamintraining.org*

Index

About the Author

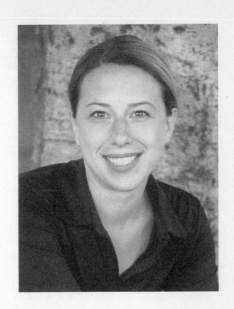

Deborah Reber is a runner, a writer and a woman (not necessarily in that order). She has been running since the seventh grade, when she took her first track steps as a sprinter. By the time she was in high school, she qualified for the Junior Olympic National Championships in the 400-meter hurdles, and was a member of the Berks County, Pennsylvania, championship cross-country team.

After a brief stint on the track team at Pennsylvania State University, Deborah turned her attention to running longer distances as a way of staying physically, and emotionally, fit. She's been a distance runner ever since. A four-time marathoner, Deborah continues to run more than a dozen road races a year, and shares her experience, insight and love for running with other women in the hopes of creating a few more addicts along the way.

Deborah recently moved from New York City to Los Angeles, where she lives with her husband, Derin, and her 13-year-old dog, Ari.